# Medical Transcription Guide

## Do's and and Don'ts

**MARILYN TAKAHASHI FORDNEY, CMA-AC, CMT**

Formerly
Instructor of Medical Insurance, Medical Terminology,
Medical Machine Transcription, and Medical Office
Procedures
Ventura College
Ventura, California

**MARCY OTIS DIEHL, BVE, CMA-A, CMT**

Instructor
Medical Typing, Medical Transcription, Medical Office
Management, Medical Terminology, Medical Insurance
Billing
Grossmont Community College
El Cajon, California

D0067671

## W.B. SAUNDERS COMPANY

*A Division of Harcourt Brace & Company*

Philadelphia   London   Toronto   Montreal   Sydney   Tokyo

**W.B. SAUNDERS COMPANY**
*A Division of*
*Harcourt Brace & Company*

The Curtis Center
Independence Square West
Philadelphia, Pennsylvania 19106

**Library of Congress Cataloging-in-Publication Data**

Fordney, Marilyn, and Diehl, Marcy
Medical Transcription Guide: Do's and Don'ts
1. Medical transcription.     I. Diehl, Marcy Otis.
II. Title. [DNLM: Medical records.     2. Medical
Secretaries.     3. Nomenclature. 80 F712m]
R728.8.F643 1990          653'.18          89-10639
ISBN 0-7216-3798-1

*Editor:*   Margaret Biblis
*Developmental Editor:*   Shirley Kuhn
*Designer:*   Joan Owen
*Production Manager:*   Carolyn Naylor
*Manuscript Editor:*   Martha Tanner
*Cover Designer:*   Anne O'Donnell

Medical Transcription Guide:
Do's and Don'ts                              ISBN   0–7216–3798–1

Copyright ©1990 by W. B. Saunders Company.

Printed in the United States of America.

Last digit is the print number:   9     8     7

# PREFACE

Welcome to *Medical Transcription Guide: Do's and Don'ts*. This book is intended for anyone who writes, types, or transcribes in the medical or scientific fields. Technology is moving at such a rapid pace that many changes have occurred in grammar and typing. Basic rules, as well as current trends and formats, are presented throughout the book. Why pick up this book rather than a standard English reference? Because in this book most of the examples provided with the rules have been chosen from medical writing, and many of these will be familiar to you from your everyday work. How many times have you had a disagreement with someone you work with on a point of grammar or punctuation in medical phrases that do not appear in English nonmedical writing? You will discover how quick and easy it is to locate the section to solve your problem. Examples of do's and don'ts allow you to see at a glance how to correct your difficulty. Rationales for specific rules are provided so you can manipulate the principles of style with knowledge and understanding.

Before you begin to use this reference, take a few minutes to glance through and see how it is organized. A detailed table of contents is provided at the beginning of the book, and each individual chapter begins with an outline for that chapter. Reference will be made to other chapters and rules when pertinent to the rule you are investigating. The book is made up of many small chapters set up in alphabetical order and titled with the key word or words that will guide you to the specific area of your research. If you cannot locate a specific topic, the surest approach is to use the index. Another feature that will grow in appeal as you familiarize yourself with the contents is the organization by rule numbers. The current rule, its exceptions, and its variations are provided along with examples and, when necessary, the common contradictions of that rule, or the *Don'ts*.

Very little narrative or explanatory material accompanies the rules, since it is assumed that the user of this book already has a working knowledge of medical typing and is either searching for help with an obscure rule or looking for reinforcement of a common practice. Some chapters will begin with an introduction to set the tone for that chapter or give you an overview of the material. It is important to read the introduction when it is provided.

Many authorities do not always agree on matters of style or grammar, so standard current practices that are generally accepted are shown as preferences, with exceptions and/or options appearing as notes following the rules. For instance, there is a trend to eliminate periods from all abbreviations. In actual fact, few writers, transcriptionists, typists, editorial boards, and journal editors act on this "modern" trend. As with all exceptions or options, you have the latitude to choose what you or your employer, the author of the material, wishes.

This book is the result of encouragement, as well as suggestions, from many medical typists who used *Medical Typing and Transcribing Techniques and Procedures* and wished for a quick reference to use on the job. We are grateful for their contributions and encourage users of this book to offer suggestions for making this handbook a more effective reference. Instructors, take note: the textbook *Medical Typing and Transcribing Techniques and Procedures* further explains and discusses many of the rules contained in this guide and provides many practical lessons for reinforcement. The third edition is available from the W.B. Saunders Company. Please write to us at the publisher's address: W.B. Saunders Company, Independence Square West, Philadelphia, PA 19106 with your comments and any constructive criticism so future editions may meet your needs.

MARILYN T. FORDNEY, CMA-AC, CMT
MARCY O. DIEHL, CMA-A, CMT

To our students, whose thirst for knowledge motivated us and in gratitude for their inspiration.

# ACKNOWLEDGMENTS

Many people have assisted in the production of this book, including our husbands, family, friends, students, former students, medical transcriptionists, and other instructors. We are especially grateful for their encouragement and help.

We appreciate those who reviewed the material and gave concrete and helpful suggestions.

Thank you to Adrienne Yazijian, CMT, and Hazel Tank, CMT, for their kind and expert advice.

We are most indebted to many individuals on the staff of the W. B. Saunders Company for their participation in making this text a reality, with special thanks to Margaret M. Biblis, Health-Related Professions Editor; Neil Litt, Supervisor, Desktop Publishing Department; Shirley Kuhn, Developmental Editor; and Martha Tanner, Copy Editor.

# CONTENTS

# 1

# ABBREVIATIONS

## AND

## SYMBOLS

## INTRODUCTION

Abbreviations are written in lower-case letters, in upper-case (capital) letters, or in a combination of upper-case and lower-case letters, with or without punctuation. Abbreviation reference books often are in conflict with one another concerning this issue. Be consistent with the guidelines that you choose. General guidelines will be offered in this chapter to assist you. A complete list of common medical abbreviations will not be provided. You should have a good abbreviation reference book available. (See Chapter 31, *Reference Materials and Publications*.)

## 1—1   ACADEMIC DEGREES, LICENSURE, RELIGIOUS ORDERS

**_DO_**  abbreviate and punctuate academic degrees and religious orders.

M.D.  Ph.D.  D.D.S.  B.V.E.  M.S.  LL.D.
S.J.  O.S.A.

**NOTE.**  *There is a strong move to eliminate the punctuation from these abbreviations, particularly in publications. Always follow the wishes of the author of the material or editorial policy of the publisher.*

**DON'T**  punctuate certification, registration, and licensure abbreviations.

CMT  RRA  ART  RN  LVN  MFCC

**_DO_**  place abbreviations for honor after academic degrees and in order of increasing distinction.

Neal J. Kaufman, M.D., FACCP

Rachel L. Connors, M.D., L.L.B.

**_DO_**  conform always to the preference of the person as far as sequence and exactly what is listed.

## 1—2   ACCURACY WITH ABBREVIATIONS

See also Rules 1–18 and 1–19 for hospital rules concerning spelling out abbreviations and accurate use of abbreviations.

**_DO_**  spell out an abbreviation when you realize that there could be a misunderstanding in its interpretation. You must be positive, of course, that _your_ interpretation is correct; otherwise, leave it alone.

The patient had a history of CVRD.

cardiovascular renal disease?
or
cardiovascular respiratory disease?

**DON'T**  spell out abbreviations that are commonly acceptable.

He was treated with Stelazine 10 mg t.i.d. with considerable improvement.

## 1—3  ACRONYMS

**_DO_**  write acronyms (a word formed from the initial letters of other words) in full capital letters without punctuation.

AIDS (_a_cquired _i_mmune _d_eficiency _s_yndrome)
CARE (_C_ooperative for _A_merican _R_emittance to _E_verywhere)
COBOL (_Co_mmon _B_usiness-_O_riented _L_anguage)
EAST (_e_xternal rotation, _a_bduction, _s_tress _t_est)
HOPE (_H_ealth _O_pportunities for _P_eople _E_verywhere)
NASA (_N_ational _A_eronautics and _S_pace _A_dministration)
NOW (_N_ational _O_rganization for _W_omen)
PERRLA (_p_upils _e_qual, _r_ound, _r_eactive to _l_ight and _a_ccommodation)
POMR (_p_roblem _o_riented _m_edical _r_ecord)
ROM (_R_ead _O_nly _M_emory)
SOAP (_s_ubjective, _o_bjective, _a_ssessment, _p_lan)
WATS (_W_ide _A_rea _T_elecommunications)
ZIP code (_Z_one _I_mprovement _P_rogram)

**DON'T**   use capital letters to write acronyms that have become accepted as words in themselves, e.g., laser, radar, scuba.

## 1—4   ADDRESS PARTS

**_DO_**   use the post office abbreviations for the state names (Fig. 1–1) on both the inside and outside addresses.

### Two-Letter State Abbreviations for the United States and Its Dependencies

| | | | | | |
|---|---|---|---|---|---|
| Alabama | AL | Kentucky | KY | Oklahoma | OK |
| Alaska | AK | Louisiana | LA | Oregon | OR |
| Arizona | AZ | Maine | ME | Pennsylvania | PA |
| Arkansas | AR | Maryland | MD | Puerto Rico | PR |
| California | CA | Massachusetts | MA | Rhode Island | RI |
| Canal Zone | CZ | Michigan | MI | South Carolina | SC |
| Colorado | CO | Minnesota | MN | South Dakota | SD |
| Connecticut | CT | Mississippi | MS | Tennessee | TN |
| Delaware | DE | Missouri | MO | Texas | TX |
| District of Columbia | DC | Montana | MT | Utah | UT |
| Florida | FL | Nebraska | NE | Vermont | VT |
| Georgia | GA | Nevada | NV | Virginia | VA |
| Guam | GU | New Hampshire | NH | Virgin Islands | VI |
| Hawaii | HI | New Jersey | NJ | Washington | WA |
| Idaho | ID | New Mexico | NM | West Virginia | WV |
| Illinois | IL | New York | NY | Wisconsin | WI |
| Indiana | IN | North Carolina | NC | Wyoming | WY |
| Iowa | IA | North Dakota | ND | | |
| Kansas | KS | Ohio | OH | | |

### Two-Letter Abbreviations for Canadian Provinces and Territories

| | | | | | |
|---|---|---|---|---|---|
| Alberta | AB | Newfoundland | NF | Quebec | PQ |
| British Columbia | BC | Northwest Territories | NT | Saskatchewan | SK |
| Labrador | LB | Nova Scotia | NS | Yukon Territory | YT |
| Manitoba | MB | Ontario | ON | | |
| New Brunswick | NB | Prince Edward Island | PE | | |

**Figure 1–1.**   United States Postal Service abbreviations for states, provinces, and territories.

936 North Branch Street
Bay Village, OH 44140

**DON'T**    abbreviate the words *street, road, avenue, boulevard, north, south, east, west* in an inside address. However, *southwest* (SW), *northwest* (NW), and so forth **are** abbreviated **after** the street name.

936 North Branch Street

1876 Washington Boulevard, NW

## 1—5    CHART NOTES AND PROGRESS NOTES

*DO*    use abbreviations freely in office chart notes and reports. Use them infrequently, except as indicated in previous rules, in formal correspondence, legal reports, articles, and hospital reports.

*Office note:* The GU tract was clear.

*Report to insurance examiner:* The genitourinary tract was clear.

*Office note:* pt had cysto on 7-1-9X

*Office consultation report to another physician:* The patient had cystoscopy performed on July l, 199X.

*Hospital history and physical report:* Patient had cystoscopy (or cysto) on 7-1-9X. (Complete sentences are not necessary.)

## 1—6    CHEMICAL AND MATH ABBREVIATIONS

**_DO_**    write chemical and mathematical abbreviations in a combination of both upper-case and lower-case letters without periods.

$CO_2$ or CO2        DNA
$T_4$ or T4          pH
$O_2$ or O2          mmHg
$Ca^{++}$            Lys
Val                  $10^4$
KCl                  Trp

**DON'T**    write these as abbreviations if the dictator has used the full word **without** a number in the expression or sentence.

There was a high *sodium* level noted. (not "a high *Na* level")

## 1—7    COMMON ABBREVIATIONS

**_DO_**    type familiar, frequently used common abbreviations, and words that can be readily understood as abbreviations, as abbreviations with no punctuation. These abbreviations usually apply to hospital departments and areas; time zones; business, educational, union, government, and military facilities; fraternal, service, professional, and religious organizations; and network and local broadcasting companies. They often represent long, complicated (forgotten?) words, or words that are seldom or never seen in any form other than an abbreviation.

DNA    ER    pH    Rh    PDR    MST    FBI    CBS
FICA    TAC    AMA    ICU    TWA    NAACP    KJQY
YMCA

## 1—8   COURTESY TITLES

**_DO_**       abbreviate and punctuate *Mrs., Mr., Dr., Ms., Jr., Sr.* when used with a surname.

> Dr. William A. Blake
> Mrs. Frances Fishbein

**_DO_**       drop the titles *Mr., Mrs., Ms., Dr.* if another title is used.

> Clifford Storey, M.D.,
> **Incorrect:** Dr. Clifford Storey, M.D.
> **Incorrect:** Dr. William A. Blake, Ph.D.

**DON'T**   abbreviate courtesy titles when used alone.

> The *doctor* was not in attendance at the time.

**DON'T**   abbreviate titles, other than *Dr., Mr., Mrs., Ms.,* **unless** a first name or initial accompanies the last name.

> Major Emery
> Honorable Wilson
> Right Reverend Turner *or* Rt. Rev. John J. Turner

## 1—9   DAYS OF THE WEEK AND MONTHS

**DON'T**   abbreviate the days of the week and months of the year. To avoid confusion, numbers should not be substituted for the names of the months in correspondence; however, the use of 6-digit dates is acceptable and often preferable in dating some records and reports.

**Correct:** January 11, 199X

**Incorrect:** Jan. 11, 199X, 1-11-9X, 01-11-9X, 1/11/9X

## 1—10    GENUS AND SPECIES

**_DO_**    abbreviate the genus (but not the species) **after** the genus has been used once in the text.

The test result was negative for Escherichia coli. We had expected to find E. coli . . .

**DON'T**    abbreviate the genus when used alone.

His Mycoplasma serology will not be repeated.

## 1—11    LATIN ABBREVIATIONS

**_DO_**    write Latin abbreviations in lower-case letters with periods.

| | |
|---|---|
| i.e. | a.c. |
| op. cit. | b.i.d. |
| et al. | t.i.d. |
| etc. | q.i.d. |
| e.g. | |
| a.m.    Also now seen as AM | |
| p.m.    Also now seen as PM | |

_EXCEPTION._    A.D. (in the year of Our Lord)

**1**

**DON'T**   insert periods inaccurately in Latin abbreviations. Check the abbreviation when in doubt.

**Incorrect:** et. al. (*et* means *and* in Latin and requires no period)

**Correct:** et al.

**DO**   avoid the overuse of Latin abbreviation substitutes for Latin phrases and replace them with the English equivalent written out.

*not* e.g.   (for *exempli gratia*)   *but*   for example

*not* etc.   (for *et cetera*)   *but*   and so forth

## 1—12   MEASUREMENTS: METRIC AND ENGLISH

**DO**   abbreviate all metric and English terms of measurement when used with a number. Use lower case letters for all but the abbreviation for liter (L) and degrees Celsius (°C) and use no punctuation marks. (**Exceptions:** *unit* and *grain*.)

20 kg   2 cm   4 oz   1000 ml   1 L   3 ft   4 in   175 lb
16 gm   7 ml or 7 mL   34°C   65 wpm   3 sq in

There was 3 oz left.
(Please notice the use of the singular form of the verb. The *three ounces* represents a single unit.)

**DON'T**   abbreviate these measurements when they are used without a number.

The cut was several *centimeters* long. (*not* cm)

# 1 ABBREVIATIONS AND SYMBOLS

**DON'T** use plural forms with measurement abbreviations.

> **Incorrect**: There *were* 3 *ozs* left.
> (The 3 ounces is seen as a single unit, so the singular verb form is also required.)

**DON'T** abbreviate *unit* or *grain*. The grain abbreviation (gr) can be mistaken for gram, and the unit abbreviation (U) can be misread, particularly when written by hand.

## 1—13    NAMES

**DON'T** abbreviate names unless the name is abbreviated in the correspondent's own letterhead. (Shortened forms of a person's name, such as a nickname, are allowed in the salutation.)

> **Incorrect:**  Chas. W. Ingles, M.D.
> Judge Bea Murphy

> **Correct:**  Judge Beatrice L. Murphy
> (followed by an informal salutation: Dear Bea,)

## 1—14    PLURAL FORMS WITH ABBREVIATIONS

***DO*** use an apostrophe to form the plurals of lower-case abbreviations and abbreviations that include periods.

M.D.'s   dsg's (dressings)   jt's (joints)

**DON'T** use an apostrophe with other plural abbreviations.

EKGs   BMRs   TMs   DTRs

## 1—15   PUNCTUATION WITH ABBREVIATIONS

**_DO_**   write most abbreviations in full capital letters without punctuation.

UCLA   PKU   BUN   CBC   WBC   COPD   D&C
NBC   FICA   TV   FM   T&A   I&C   P&A   JFK

**DON'T**   punctuate most abbreviations written in a combination of upper- and lower-case letters.

Rx   Dx   ACh   Ba   Hb   IgG   mEq   mOsm

**_DO_**   use a period and space between the initial and the name following the initial.

William A. Knox Jr.

**DON'T**   use a comma between *Jr.* or *Sr.* and the surname.

*NOTE.   This is the current trend. Always follow the dictates of the person if he prefers otherwise.*

**DON'T**   use a comma between *II, III, 2d, 3d,* etc., and the surname.

William A. Knox II

*NOTE.   This is the current trend. Always follow the dictates of the person if he prefers otherwise.*

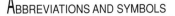
## 1—16    SAINT, ABBREVIATED

**_DO_**    abbreviate and punctuate *Saint* (St.) when it is the name of a place or part of the name of a person who prefers the abbreviation.

Margaret St. James

St. Paul, Minnesota

## 1—17    SENTENCE STRUCTURE

**DON'T**    begin a sentence with an abbreviation. Restructure the sentence or spell out the abbreviation.

## 1—18    SHORT FORMS

**_DO_**    type the short forms, or brief forms, when dictated if they do not violate any of the guidelines listed under Rule 1–19.

Pap smear (Papanicolaou)
exam (examination)
sed rate (sedimentation rate)
flu (influenza)
phenobarb (phenobarbital)

## 1—19    SPELLED-OUT ABBREVIATONS

**_DO_**    use an abbreviation to refer to a test, committee, drug, diagnosis, and so forth in a report or paper *after* it has been used once in its completely spelled-out form.

All newborns are routinely tested for phenylketonuria (PKU). As a result, the incidence of PKU as a cause of infant . . .

*NOTE. Some abbreviations, particularly acronyms, become so common that it is no longer necessary to spell out the meaning.*

It took a long time for the public to respond to the AIDS crisis.

**DO**      spell out all abbreviations in the admission and discharge diagnoses, preoperative and postoperative diagnoses, impressions, assessments, and the names of surgical procedures.

Discharge diagnosis: Pelvic inflammatory disease
*(not PID)*

Operation performed: Tonsillectomy and
adenoidectomy
*(not T&A)*

**DON'T**      use symbols and abbreviations in the medical record when they have not been approved and listed by the medical staff. These lists will vary among institutions.

**DO**      avoid using abbreviations in the titles of abstracts and papers or articles for publication.

## 1—20    STATE NAMES

**DO**      use the two-letter state abbreviations approved by the United States Postal Service for both inside and envelope addresses (see Figure 1–1).

# 1 ABBREVIATIONS AND SYMBOLS

**DON'T**    use the abbreviations without the city name and ZIP code.

## 1—21 SYMBOLS WITH ABBREVIATIONS

Symbols are just another form of abbreviation. Most standard symbols are available on the typewriter and word processing font menus.

***DO***    use the ampersand symbol (&) with abbreviations.

I&D   P&A   L&W

***DO***    use symbols only when they occur in immediate association with a number or another abbreviation.

| | |
|---|---|
| $8 \times 3$ | eight by three |
| $4-5$ | four to five |
| #3−0 | number three oh |
| 2+ | two plus |
| Vision: 20/20 | vision is twenty-twenty |
| 6/day | six per day |
| diluted 1:10 | diluted one to ten |
| at −2 | at minus two |
| 60/40 | sixty over forty |
| nocturia $\times 2$ | nocturia times two |
| T&A | tonsillectomy and adenoidectomy |
| 25 mg/hr | twenty-five milligrams per hour |
| limited by 45% | limited by forty-five percent |
| 35 mg/dl | thirty-five milligrams per deciliter |
| 30° C | thirty degrees Celsius |
| 99° F | ninty-nine degrees Fahrenheit |
| BP: 100/80 | blood pressure is one hundred over eighty |
| rSR´ | RSR prime |

**DO**    spell out the symbol abbreviation when it is used alone, not in association with a number.

What is the *percentage* of cure rates using this modality? (not %)

## 1—22    TITLES

**DO**    use the abbreviation *Esq.* **only** when no other title is used.

D. Kirk Knight, Esq.
**Incorrect:** Mr. D. Kirk Knight, Esq.

*NOTE.    The spelled-out* Esquire *is also correct.*

**DO**    drop the titles *Mr., Mrs., Ms., Dr.* if another title is used.

Clifford Storey, M.D.
**Incorrect:** Dr. Clifford Storey, M.D.

**DO**    use any required punctuation mark, except a period, after the period used with an abbreviation.

Are you sure his name is John R. Robertson Sr.?

The topics in this chapter are not arranged alphabetically but rather in the progression of an address from top to bottom, i.e., from name of addressee to salutation and finishing with the complete address.

# 2

# ADDRESS

# FORMATS

# FOR LETTERS

# AND FORMS

# OF ADDRESS

# Address Formats for Letters

## INTRODUCTION

The inside address is typed flush with the left margin and is begun on approximately the fifth line below the date of the letter. It may be moved up or down one line depending on the length of the letter.

## 2—1    NAMES OF PERSONS AND FIRMS

A courtesy or professional title is added to a name. If you do not know whether the person is a man or a woman, omit using a title. The title "Ms." may be used when you do not have a title for a woman. The degree is preferred over a title, and in no case should a title and a degree be used together. Use the middle initial when it is known.

**DON'T**    use both title and degree with a name.

*Incorrect:*
Dr. Clifford F. Adolph, M.D.
Dr. Bertrum L. Storey, D.D.S
Mrs. Beatrice Wood, Ph.D.

*Correct:*
Dr. Beatrice Wood
Beatrice Wood, Ph.D.
Mrs. Beatrice Wood (in a social setting)

***DO***    use the complete name of a person with courtesy title.

Ms. Mary T. Jordan
Professor Otis R. Laban
Drs. Reilly, Lombardo and Chesney
Dora F. Hodge, M.D.
Captain Denis K. Night
Glenn M. Stempen, D.D.S. or Dr. Glenn M. Stempen
Miss Rita B. Reed-Winthrop

**DON'T**     abbreviate any part of the name unless the person does so on his letterhead.

William A. Berry, M.D. *not* Wm. A. Berry, M.D.

*DO*     copy the complete name of the firm exactly as it is printed on the letterhead or as printed in the telephone book or other professional directory. Always follow the firm's style for capitalization, abbreviations, and punctuation.

Palm Grove Medical Center
South Bay Medical Group Ltd.
Atlantic Shores 24-Hour Clinic
Valley Presbyterian Hospital
Maynard County Medical Supply
Mountain States Instrument Company Inc.
Lake Shore County Dental Society
Kimbrell, Owen, Sweis & Schonbrun

**DON'T**     use a comma to set off *Inc., Ltd.*, and so forth from the company name unless the company does so.

*DO*     place abbreviations for honor and academic degrees after the name and in order of increasing distinction.

Neal J. Kaufman, M.D., FACCP
Rachel L. Connors, M.D., L.L.B.

*NOTE.     There is a current trend to eliminate the period punctuation mark from all degree symbols. Always use the method acceptable to your employer or to the editorial staff when preparing a document for publication.*

*DO*     separate the parts of a name with a comma or commas when it is given in inverted order.

Jacobs, Barney K.
Kaufman, Neal J., M.D., FACP

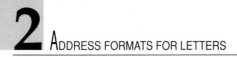

# 2 ADDRESS FORMATS FOR LETTERS

## 2—2   TITLES

If a business title accompanies the name, it may follow the name on the same line, or, if lengthy, it may appear on the next line. When two lines are used, no punctuation is placed at the end of the first line and the title is typed flush with the name above

**_DO_**   use titles when and as appropriate.

F.E. Gidwani, M.D., Medical Director

Ms. Catherine A. Wendall
Purchasing Agent

Adrian N. Abott, M.D., L.L.B.
Chief-of-Staff
Sinai-Lebanon Hospital

Dean Karl T. Brent, Chairman
Biology Department
International University

## 2—3   ADDRESS

Following the name of the person or firm is the street or post office box address. (If both are given, use the post office box address.) Abbreviations are printed after the street name only (see Rule 1–4). They include NW, NE, SW, and so forth. Do not abbreviate North, South, East, West, Road, Street, Avenue, or Boulevard. "Apartment" is abbreviated only if the line is unusually long. The apartment, suite, or space number is typed on the same line with the street address, separated by a comma.

The name of the city is spelled out and separated from the state name with a comma. The state name may be spelled out or abbreviated and is separated from the ZIP code by one to three spaces. The United States postal abbreviations are not used without the ZIP code (see Rule 1–20).

***DO***     complete the address as approved by United States postal regulations, avoiding all unnecessary abbreviations. For ease of understanding, spell out the number *one* when it is the street, building, or apartment number.

| | |
|---|---|
| One Cable Avenue<br>Little Creek, CA 94524 | P.O. Box 1966<br>Naples, FL 33940 |
| 1731 North Branch Road, Suite B<br>Toledo, OH 43505 | P.O. Box 17433, Foy Station<br>Chicago, IL 60636 |
| 845 Medford Circle, Apartment 54<br>Bearden, KS 66743 | Rural Route #3<br>Crow Poison, AK 99516 |

196 Blackmoor Road
Hatchend
Pinner, Middlesex
ENGLAND HA 5 4PF

**DON'T**     use post office abbreviations without the ZIP code.

# Forms of Address/Salutations

## INTRODUCTION

   The manner in which a person is addressed in a letter is determined by the relationship between the writer and the receiver of the document, if the receiver is known. If the receiver of the document is unknown, careful protocol must be observed and stereotypic language avoided.

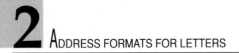

**Placement and Punctuation of Salutation:** The salutation is typed a double space after the last line of the address and is followed by a colon if mixed punctuation is used. If open punctuation is used, neither a colon nor comma is utilized. Formality demands a courtesy title; first names are used when appropriate and if formality is unnecessary.

## 2—4 SALUTATIONS USED FOR MEN

***DO***      follow these formats when addressing men:

Gentlemen:

Dear Mr. Sutherland:

Dear Dr. Hon: *(or)*
Dear Doctor Hon:

Dear Drs. Blake and Fortuna:
Dear Dr. Blake and Dr. Fortuna:
Dear Doctors:
Dear Paul and Josh: *or* Dear Paul and Josh,

***NOTE.*** *When using first names only, a comma is also correct.*

Dear Dr. Johnson and Mr. Lombardo:
Gentlemen:
Dear Chuck and Jay:
Dear Chuck and Jay,

Dear Professor Abbott:
Dear Dr. Abbott:

Dear Rabbi Ruderman:
(likewise Father, Bishop, Reverend, Monsignor, Cardinal, Brother, Deacon, Chaplain, Dean)

Dear Mr. Tony Lamb and Mr. Peter Lamb:
Dear Messrs. Lamb:
Gentlemen:
Dear Tony and Pete:
Dear Tony and Pete,

## 2—5  SALUTATIONS USED FOR WOMEN

**_DO_**  follow these formats when addressing women:

Ladies:
Mesdames:

Dear Dr. Martin:
Dear Doctor Martin:

Dear Mrs. Clayborne:

Dear Ms. Robinson:

Dear Miss Glenn:

Dear Judge Peterson:

Dear Rev. Schwartz:
(likewise Rabbi, Chaplain, Dean, Deacon, Bishop)

Dear Sister Rose Anthony:

Dear Reverend Mother Reilly:
Dear Reverend Mother:

Dear Captain Jenkins:

Dear Professor Mayz:

Dear Dr. Rose Martin and Dr. Lily Martin:
Dear Drs. Martin:
Dear Doctors:
Dear Rose and Lily:
Dear Rose and Lily,

Dear Drs. Person and Higgins:
Dear Dr. Person and Dr. Higgins:
Dear Doctors:
Dear Jeanette and Beverly:
Dear Jeanette and Beverly,

Dear Dr. Phillips and Ms. Cox:
Ladies:
Dear Bertha and Wanda:
Dear Bertha and Wanda,

Dear Mses. Ostrom and Allen:
Dear Mrs. Ostrom and Mrs. Allen:
Ladies:
Dear Irma and Bobbie:
Dear Irma and Bobbie,

Dear Mrs. Heaney and Ms. Heaney:
Ladies:
Dear Kristen and Andrea:
Dear Kristen and Andrea,

**DON'T**    Use social titles in business correspondence:

*Incorrect:*
Dear *Mrs. John Becker* and Ms. Patty Becker:

*Correct:*
Dear *Mrs. Sheila Becker* and Ms. Patty Becker:
Ladies:
Dear Sheila and Patty:
Dear Sheila and Patty,

## 2—6 FORMATS FOR ADDRESSING MEN AND WOMEN AS A MARRIED COUPLE

**_DO_**  follow these formats when addressing men and women as a married couple:

Dear Mr. and Mrs. Knight:

Dear Dr. and Mrs. Wong:
Dear Doctor and Mrs. Wong:

Dear Professor and Mrs. Barnett:

Dear Professor Holloway and Ms. Blake:

Dear Professor and Mr. Collings:

Dear Dr. Johnson and Ms. Lombardo:

Dear Rabbi Gold and Mr. Gold:
Dear Lila and Bob:
Dear Lila and Bob,

Dear Dr. Lois Candelaria and Dr. Fred Candelaria:
Dear Drs. Candelaria:
Dear Doctors:
Dear Lois and Fred:

Dear Captain and Mrs. Philips:

Dear Mr. Claborne and Mrs. Steen-Claborne:

Dear Mr. Mohrman and Captain Mohrman:

Dear Mr. Bailey and Dr. Bailey:
Dear Dr. and Mr. Bailey:

## 2—7 FORMATS FOR ADDRESSING MEN AND WOMEN
NOT ASSOCIATED AS A MARRIED COUPLE

**_DO_**

follow these formats when addressing men and women who are not associated as a married couple

Dear Drs. DuPree and Ahrens:
Dear Dr. DuPree and Dr. Ahrens:
Dear Doctors:
Dear Nancy and Philip:

Dear Dr. Cleveland and Mrs. Easterly:
Dear Dr. Cleveland and Ms. Easterly:
Dear Patrick and Connie:

Dear Professor Garcia and Mr. Ireton:

Dear Professor Kimbrell and Ms. Knudsen:

## 2—8 FORMATS FOR ADDRESSING LARGE GROUPS
OF MEN AND/OR WOMEN

**_DO_**

follow this format when addressing a large group of men and/or women:

Gentlemen:
Ladies and Gentlemen:
Ladies:
Dear Doctors:

Dear Professor Bradley et al.:
Dear Dr. Mitchelson et al.: (*use just the name of the senior person in the firm.*)

## 2—9    FORMATS FOR ADDRESSING UNKNOWN GENDER OR UNKNOWN RECIPIENT

**DON'T**    assign gender to the head of a firm.

*DO*    follow these formats when the gender is unknown:

Ladies and Gentlemen:
Dear Sir or Madam:

Dear Lane Wilkerson:

*DO*    follow this format when the recipient of the document is unknown:

To Whom It May Concern:
TO WHOM IT MAY CONCERN:

## 2—10    ATTENTION LINE

The attention line is typed two spaces below the last line of the address. It is used so that the letter will receive attention by a specific person if he or she is available; if not, another member of the firm will take care of the matter.

*DO*    type *attention* in full caps or with only the first letter capitalized.

ATTENTION ~~Mr.~~ Charles P. Trask, Buyer *or*
Attention Mr. Charles P. Trask, Buyer

**DON'T**   abbreviate *Attention* or use punctuation with it.

ATTN: Mr. Charles P. Trask, Buyer (incorrect)

*DO*   type an appropriate salutation with an attention line. Since the first line of the address is the firm name, the salutation must be in keeping with **this** line rather than the attention line. The following salutations are appropriate:

Dear Sir or Madam:

Gentlemen:

Ladies:

Ladies and Gentlemen:

Doctors:

Dear Doctors:

*NOTE.*   *Many secretaries find it awkward to follow an attention line that is obviously addressed to a specific person with a non-specific salutation. For example:*

Engraved Letterhead Company
2171 Lincoln Boulevard
Philadelphia, PA 19105

ATTENTION Pauline Flinn, Buyer

Dear Sir or Madam:

*However, this example is correct. It is suggested that one might address this document instead directly to Ms. Flinn and omit the Attention Line, so that the saluation then would read* Dear Ms. Flinn.

## 2—11   COMPLETE ADDRESS APPEARANCE

**_DO_**   strive to prepare an attractive, balanced inside address. If one line is significantly longer than the rest, find an appropriate dividing point on the long line.

Victor R. Langworthy, M.D.
Medical Director
West View Community Hospital and Inland Medical Center, Inc.
321 Roseview Drive
St. Louis, MO 63139

*better arrangement*:

Victor R. Langworthy, M.D., Medical Director
West View Community Hospital and
   Inland Medical Center, Inc.
32l Roseview Drive
St. Louis, MO 63139

Miss Josie M. Brooks
1879 Westchester Boulevard, Apartment 170-B
Normal Heights, SD 57701

*better arrangement*:

Miss Josie M. Brooks
Apartment 170-B
1879 Westchester Boulevard
Normal Heights, SD 57701

**_DO_**   type each name on a separate line when you are preparing a letter to more than one individual.

William A. Blake, M.D.
Ralph P. Fortuna, M.D.
Street address
City, State + ZIP

Peter L. Johnson, D.D.S.
Mr. Frank R. Lombardo
Street address
City, State + ZIP

Mr. Tony Lamb
Mr. Peter Lamb
Street address
City, State + ZIP

Rose Q. Martin, M.D.
Lily A. Martin, M.D.
Street address
City, State + ZIP

Renee L. Phillips, D.O.
Ms. Francine T. Cox
Street address
City, State + ZIP

Mrs. Sally B. Ostrom
Mrs. Sharon R. Allen
Street address
City, State + ZIP

Lois Jean Candelaria, M.D.
Fred P. Candelaria, Ph.D.
Street address
City, State + ZIP

Mrs. Glendora Robinson
c/o Steven Santiago
Street address
City, State + ZIP

Drs. Mitchelson, Francois, Peters, Moore, & Davis
Street Address
City, State + ZIP

Dear Dr. Mitchelson et al.:

# 3

# APOSTROPHE

## 3—1   COMPOUND NOUNS

**_DO_**   add an apostrophe *s* to the last element of the possessive compound.

the chief-of-staff's decision
my brother-in-law's surgery

## 3—2   CONTRACTIONS

**_DO_**   use an apostrophe in contractions of words or figures.

| | |
|---|---|
| it's | (it is *or* it has) |
| he'll | (he will) |
| won't | (will not) |
| class of '91 | (1991) |
| o'clock | (of the clock) |
| I'm | (I am) |
| you're | (you are) |
| let's | (let us) |

# 3 APOSTROPHE

> **NOTE.** *With the exception of o'clock, which is always written as a contraction, use of contractions in writing should be avoided.*

## 3—3  EPONYMS

Eponyms are adjectives derived from a proper noun.

**DO**   use the rules as stated to form the possessive of eponyms that refer to parts of the anatomy, diseases, signs, or syndromes.

*Signs and Tests:*
Romberg's sign
Hoffmann's reflex
Babinski's sign
Ayer's test

*Anatomy:*
Bartholin's glands
Beale's ganglion
Mauthner's membrane

*Diseases and Syndromes:*
Fallot's tetralogy
Tietze's syndrome
Hirschsprung's disease

**DON'T**   show possession for eponyms that describe surgical instruments.

*Instruments:*
Mayo scissors
Richards retractors
Foley catheter
Liston–Stille forceps

*DO*     **when writing for publication,** substitute the specific descriptive term for a disease for the equivalent eponymic term. Further, if the author prefers the eponym, **avoid** using the possessive form. Different rules apply when writing for publication.

*Preferred:* alopecia parvimaculata syndrome
*Second choice:* Dreuw syndrome
*Not:* Dreuw's syndrome

*Preferred:* pancreatic exocrine insufficiency syndrome
*Second choice:* Clarke-Hadefield syndrome

## 3—4    JOINT POSSESSION

*DO*     show possession with the last noun when two or more nouns share possession.

Clark and Clark's new reference book is in.

Dr. Franklin and Dr. Meadow's patient was just admitted.

**DON'T**     use this rule when possession is not shared.

Dr. Franklin's and Dr. Meadow's **patients were** just admitted.

## 3—5    MISCELLANEOUS APOSTROPHE USE

*DO*     use an apostrophe when necessary to help clarify meaning.

The long convalescence was a result of Ron's falling.
She was in no mood for "what for's."
She OK'd my vacation.
He is a patient of Bob's.

**_DO_**  use the apostrophe as the symbol for the word
"prime" in completing the description of an EKG's
smaller R wave component, rSR´ (pronounced "RSR
prime"). (The lower-case "r" refers to the smaller R
wave component.)

## 3—6 PLURAL FORMS OF LETTERS AND ABBREVIATIONS

**_DO_**  use an apostrophe to form the plural of the capital let-
ters *A, I, O, M, U* and all **lower-case** single letters.

When you make an entry in the chart, be careful that
your 2s don't look like z's

Spell that with three r's.

You used four I's in the first paragraph.

**_DO_**  use an apostrophe to form the plurals and possessives
of lower-case abbreviations and abbreviations that include periods (see Rule 1–14).

There were elevated wbc's.
It was the M.D.'s decision.

**DON'T**  use the apostrophe to form the plural of numbers or
capital letter abbreviations.

The TMs were intact.
There were no 4 × 4s left in the box.

## 3—7    PLURAL POSSESSIVE NOUNS

**_DO_**     add an apostrophe *s* to plural forms of nouns.

women's studies
children's ward
mice's tracks

**_DO_**     use an apostrophe after the *s* in plural nouns that end
in *s*.

the typists' responsibility (more than one typist)
the Joneses' records (more than one Jones)
the heroes' methods
the berries' ripeness
the employees' records

**DON'T**    use an apostrophe to show possession of institutions
or organizations **unless they elect to do so.**

Veterans Administration Hospital*
Childrens Hospital
St. Josephs Infirmary
Boys Club

*and certainly not Veteran's Hospital!*

## 3—8    PRONOUNS

**_DO_**     form the possessive of relative pronouns such as
everyone, nobody, someone, anyone, and anybody,
just as you would with possessive nouns.

It is nobody's fault.
That is anyone's guess.
It is somebody else's responsibility.

# 3 APOSTROPHE

**DON'T** use an apostrophe with personal pronouns such as *its,\* hers, yours, his, theirs, ours, whose,\** or *yours.*

The next appointment is her's. (incorrect)
The dog injured it's foot. (incorrect)
You're coat is soiled. (incorrect)

*\*Notice these contractions, however:*

**It's** *time for your next appointment.*
**Who's** *going to clean the operatory?*

**COMMENT.** *Probably one of the most common errors made concerns the misuse of the apostrophe with* **it.** *Since* its *and* it's *are both correct when used in the proper context, writers often make an improper choice.*

## 3—9   SINGULAR POSSESSIVE NOUNS

**DO** use an apostrophe *s* with a singular noun not ending in *s* to show possession

the typist's responsibility (one typist)
Bob's doctor
Dr. Mitch's office

**DO** use an apostrophe only (no *s*) to show possession of singular nouns that end in *s* or in a strong *s* sound.

the waitress' table
for appearance' sake
Mr. Gomez' surgery

**DO** use an apostrophe only after the *s* in two-syllable singular proper nouns ending in *s*.

*Preferred style:*
Frances' report
Mr. Walters' point of view

*Alternate style:*
Frances's report
Mr. Walters's point of view

**DON'T** break up a proper noun that ends in an *s* by placing the apostrophe in front of the *s*.

*Concerning Mr. Walters:*
Mr. Walter's point of view (incorrect)
Mr. Walters' point of view (correct)

*DO* add an apostrophe *s* to singular nouns ending in *s* or an *s* sound when they are of a single syllable.

Mr. Jones's medical record
James Rose's appointment

## 3—10    TIME, DISTANCE, VALUE, AND SOURCE

*DO* use an apostrophe to show possession of time, distance, value, and source.

return in one month's time
at 10 weeks' gestation
get your money's worth
within a hair's breadth of injury
too much exposure to the sun's rays

**DON'T**   show possession of inanimate things.

the roof of the car *rather than* the car's roof
the color of the bruise *rather than* the bruise's color
the cover of the book *rather than* the book's cover

## 3—11   UNDERSTOOD NOUNS

***DO***   follow the same rules for showing possession when the noun is understood.

That stethoscope is Dr. Green's. (stethoscope)
He bought that at William's. (store)

I consulted Dorland's. (dictionary)
That is where he earned his master's. (degree)

# 4

# Capitalization

## 4—1    ABBREVIATIONS

**_DO_**    capitalize abbreviations when the words they represent are capitalized. Capitalize most abbreviations of English words. (See Chapter 1 for specific capitalization of abbreviations.)

ECG and EKG are both abbreviations for "electrocardiogram."

James A. Smith, M.D., graduated from UCSD.

**DO**      capitalize each letter in an acronym.

Dr. Bowman is working with Project HOPE and UNICEF.

**DON'T**      capitalize metric and English forms of measurement or Latin abbreviations. (See Rules 1–11 and 1–12.)

e.g.   t.i.d.   ft   cm   mL   oz   mph

**DO**      capitalize and punctuate the abbreviations of academic degrees.

M.D.   Ph.D.   D.D.S.   M.S.   D.O.

## 4—2   ACADEMIC COURSE NAMES

**DO**      capitalize the names of specific academic courses.

**DON'T**      capitalize academic subject areas unless they contain a proper noun.

I am enrolled in Medical Transcription 103; I am also taking anatomy and business English.

## 4—3   ALLERGIES

**DO**      draw attention to drug and food allergies by typing or writing them in full capital letters, underlining them (in black or red), emphasizing them with a highlight pen, or typing them in boldface in medical reports and chart notes.

The patient has a history of an ALLERGY TO PENICILLIN AND CODEINE PRODUCTS.

The patient has a history of an allergy to penicillin and codeine products.

The patient has a history of an **allergy to penicillin and codeine products**.

The patient denied having any food, environmental, or drug allergies.

*NOTE. Some facilities also use bright adhesive labels placed on patients' file folders to draw attention to allergies.*

## 4—4   CALENDAR AND DATES

*DO*

capitalize the names of the days of the week, months of the year, holidays, historic events and religious festivals.

There will be no class on Friday, November 11, because it is Veterans' Day.

We plan to celebrate Medical Transcriptionists' Week.

Do we get an Easter holiday or a Passover vacation? Neither, it's called "Spring Vacation."

**DON'T**

capitalize the seasons of the year.

I am taking an advanced terminology class in the spring semester; I wish I had taken it this fall.

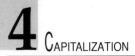

## 4—5    DEPARTMENTS AND SECTIONS IN INSTITUTIONS

**_DO_**    capitalize the names of **specific** departments or sections in the hospital or institution.

> Admitting Office
> Medical Records Department
> Childrens Wing
> Intensive Care Unit

The patient was first seen in Valley Presbyterian Hospital Emergency Room on July 1.

The Department of Surgery received the notice.

BUT

All surgery departments received the notice.

The patient was sent to the recovery room.

pathology report
operating room team

## 4—6 DISEASES AND SYNDROMES

**DO**    Capitalize only a proper name or eponym in the name of a disease or syndrome.

Down's syndrome
German measles
chickenpox
Hansen's disease
myasthenia gravis
hyaline membrane disease
San Joaquin Valley fever
Mycobacterium tuberculosis *also* M. tuberculosis
tuberculosis
Parkinson's disease
influenza *or* flu
Spanish influenza
Hemophilus influenzae

## 4—7 DRUG NAMES

**DO**    capitalize the trade names and brand names of drugs and other trademarked materials. Maintain any idiosyncratic capitalization used by the proprietor of the brand name.

**DON'T**    capitalize generic names.

**Trade names of drugs and suture materials:**
Nitora, Darvon, Cortisporin, Theokin,
pHisoHex, Gelfoam, Surgicel, Dermalon,
GoLYTELY, HydroDIURIL

**Generic names of drugs and suture materials:**
nitroglycerin, analgesic, hydrocortisone, potassium iodide, alcohol, ether, silk, catgut

**DON'T** capitalize the common noun following the brand name of a drug.

Tylenol tablets
Neosporin ointment

*NOTE. Some drug names have identical brand name and generic name spelling. Be consistent in choosing to use upper-case or lower-case letters.*

She is on Tedral, SSKI drops, Choledyl, and Prednisone.
(Prednisone can be generic or brand. Since the other drugs referred to are brand name drugs, it can be assumed that this drug is being referred to by brand name as well.)

## 4—8 GENUS AND SPECIES

*DO* capitalize the name of the genus but not the name of the species that follows it. Capitalize the name of the genus when it is written alone.

The patient was admitted by the ophthalmologist because of infection with Onchocerca volvulus.

Ralph saw the doctor because he had a bad reaction to Cannabis.

*NOTE. The genus may be referred to by its first initial only; this is capitalized with a period and followed by the species name. (See Rule 1–10.)*

E. coli (Escherichia coli)
M. tuberculosis (Mycobacterium tuberculosis)
H. influenzae (Hemophilus influenzae)

## 4—9   GEOGRAPHIC LOCATIONS

**_DO_**

capitalize both the noun and the adjective when they make reference to a **specific** geographic location.

The patient was born and raised in the Southwest; he has lived in the Deep South only a short while.

We plan to stay at a resort by the Atlantic Ocean when we go east for the medical meeting this fall.

| | |
|---|---|
| the Great Lakes | Apache Reservation |
| Cape of Good Hope | Crow Poison Crossing |

**DON'T**

capitalize the names of places when they appear before the names of a specific place or are general directions.

travel west on Highway 10
the state of New York (*but*) New York State

**_DO_**

capitalize *boulevard, street, avenue, drive, way*, and so on, when used with a proper noun.

321 Westvillage Drive

One of the most attractive streets in Naples is Palm Avenue.

## 4—10 LETTER PARTS

**DO** capitalize the first word of the salutation and the complimentary close.

Dear Dr. Reynolds:
Sincerely yours,
Yours very truly,

**DO** capitalize the first letter or all of the letters in the word *attention* when it is part of an address; capitalize the first letter of each word or all the letters in the title *To Whom It May Concern*. (See Rules 2–9 and 2–10.)

ATTENTION Reservation Clerk
*or*
Attention Reservation Clerk

TO WHOM IT MAY CONCERN:
*or*
To Whom It May Concern:

**DO** capitalize a person's title in business correspondence when it appears in the inside address, typed signature, line, or envelope address.

Ms. Marilyn Alan, President
W. Raul Deal, M.D., Director
ATTENTION Ralph Cavanaugh, Buyer

**DO** capitalize both letters of the state abbreviation when it is part of the address and precedes the ZIP code. (See Figure 1–1, p. 4.)

District Heights, MD 20028
San Diego, CA 92119

**_DO_**    capitalize names, proper nouns, well-known nick-names for proper nouns, adjectives derived from proper nouns, and eponyms.

Josephine Holman just moved here from the Rockies and is looking for a job as a medical secretary.

We learned that valley fever is endemic to Imperial Valley, San Joaquin Valley, and the Sonoran deserts.

Sometimes I think he's more Hoosier than American.

**Eponyms:**
I am afraid that the diagnosis is Hodgkin's disease.
We need a #15 Foley catheter.

**DON'T**    capitalize the following eponyms, which are exceptions to this general rule and have acquired independent common meaning.

| | |
|---|---|
| arabic numbers | manila folder |
| braille symbol | mendelian genetics |
| cesarean section | paris green |
| chinese blue | parkinsonism* |
| curie unit | pasteurized milk |
| cushingoid signs | petri dish |
| epsom salt | plaster of paris |
| eustachian tube | portland cement |
| fallopian tube | roentgen unit |
| french fries | roman numeral |
| india ink | siamese twins |
| kleig light | |

*NOTE. See Chapter 12, Eponyms, for complete use of eponyms.*

*\*but Parkinson's disease.*

# 4 CAPITALIZATION

**_DO_**     capitalize the official names of organizations, publications, conferences, governmental agencies, symposia, postgraduate courses, and so forth.

American College of Chest Physicians
Pima County Medical Society
Sports Medicine and Rehabilitation
Board of Medical Quality Assurance
Medical Political Action Committee
United States Navy
American Medical Association

**DON'T**     capitalize the article *the* in referring to newspapers and magazines.

the Wall Street Journal

**DON'T**     capitalize the prefix in hyphenated proper nouns but do capitalize the proper noun that follows it.

non-Hodgkins          mid-May
anti-Semitic          pseudo-Christian
anti-American
ex-President Franklin

*EXCEPTION:*   Pre-Raphaelite

**_DO_**     capitalize all references to a Supreme Being.

God            Messiah          Holy Spirit
Allah          Lord of All      Son of God
Mother Nature                   the Almighty

## 4—12  NUMBERS WITH NOUNS

**_DO_**     capitalize nouns that are closely associated with and immediately precede numbers.

>  We ordered a Model 14 Medtronic pacemaker.
>  He has a Grade II systolic murmur.
>  You have a reservation on Flight 707.

**DON'T**  capitalize the following common exceptions to the rule: page number, paragraph, line, sentence, note, and size.

>  There is an error in your copy on page 27, paragraph 2, line 3.

## 4—13  OUTLINES AND LISTS

**_DO_**     capitalize the first word of each line in an outline or list.

>  Diagnoses:     1. Stress incontinence of urine.
>                          2. Monilial vaginitis.

**_DO_**     use full caps for the major and minor headings in reports. Major headings may be underlined. (See Chapter 19, _Medical Reports,_ for complete report formats.)

>  HEENT:
>  HEAD: Normal.
>  EYES: Pupils round and equal, react to L&A.
>  EARS: Hearing normal, TMs intact, canals patent.

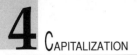

# 4 Capitalization

## 4—14 RACES AND PEOPLES

**_DO_**    capitalize the names of races, peoples, religions, and languages.

He is a well-developed, well-nourished, Oriental businessman in no acute distress.

The patient is a 59-year-old Caucasian female oriented to time, place, and person.

She is a Catholic, but they decided to be married in the Jewish temple.

We are taking an evening course in medical Spanish because we have many Hispanic patients who do not speak English.

**DON'T**    capitalize the words white or black when they are used to describe a race.

## 4—15 SENTENCES AND QUOTATIONS

**_DO_**    capitalize the first word of the sentence, the first word of a complete direct quotation, and the first word after a colon **if** that word begins a complete thought.

The instructor said, "Strive for mailable copy even when you are practice-typing."

She told him to "strive for perfection."

These are your directions: Begin typing as soon as you hear the signal, and stop when the timer rings.

Diagnosis: Acute cervical strain.

**DON'T**    begin a sentence with a number written as a figure or with an abbreviation.

## 4—16    TITLES, FAMILY

**_DO_**    capitalize a title that designates a member of the family **unless** it is preceded by a possessive noun or pronoun.

My father is bringing Aunt Mary here this afternoon for her flu shot.

The patient's mother died of carcinoma of the breast at age 56, and his father is living and well.

I saw Dad only last week.
I saw my dad last week.

**DON'T**    capitalize a title when it is followed by an appositive.

My uncle, William Peters, moved here recently from Cleveland.

## 4—17    TITLES, LITERARY

**_DO_**    capitalize the first and last words and all other words in the titles of articles, books, and periodicals, with the exception of conjunctions, prepositions, or articles.

# 4 Capitalization

**DON'T** capitalize locants or other chemical prefixes and uncapitalized taxonomic names in a title.

The title of the film is "Unusual Reactions to the Use of Cannabis sativa."

The working title of the paper is "Isomer 11-cis-Retinal Rod Combination Factors."

*NOTE.* *Major literary works are also underlined; minor ones are enclosed in quotation marks.*

Do you use the reference <u>The Medical Word Book</u> by Sheila Sloane?

He is slated to read his paper "Just a Few Beers?" at the next medical society meeting.

**_DO_** capitalize only the initial letter in first word, proper nouns, scientific names, and the initial letters of abbreviated journal titles in a bibliographic reference.

Dodd JS, ed. <u>The ACS Style Guide: A Manual for Authors and Editors.</u> Washington: American Chemical Society; 1986.

Stromgren BJ. Voice recognition: a new technique for operative reporting. J. Am. Med. Rec. Assoc. Feb 1988; 59:20–22.

## 4—18   TITLES, ORGANIZATIONAL

**_DO_**   capitalize the titles of organizations and the titles of officers in an organization's minutes, bylaws, or rules.

The Secretary read the minutes, and they were approved as read.

Dr. Sanderson has recently retired from the Navy.

The President proposed that the Board of Directors be polled.

American Cancer Society
Knights of Columbus
Toastmaster, Inc.
Eastridge Clinic
United States Air Force

## 4—19   TITLES, PERSONAL AND PROFESSIONAL

**_DO_**   capitalize a person's title in business correspondence when it appears in the inside address, typed signature line, or envelope address.

Jean Lusk, M.D., Chief-of-Staff
Rhonda Williams, Dean
Charles Bruno, CMT, Secretary

**_DO_**    capitalize military, political, and professional titles
when they immediately **precede** the name.

Capt. Max Draper
Dr. Ralph P. Smith
President Fernando Morales
Dean Caldwell
Monsignor Rayfield
Rabbi Hinz

Dr. Randolph is president of the medical society.

The attorney will be here at 9:30 to meet with the doctor about his testimony.

She is taking the examination to become a certified medical transcriptionist.

*NOTE.   Only titles of high distinction are capitalized **following** a person's name, except in the address and typed signature line. "High distinction" can be very subjective, depending upon who is doing the writing. "High distinction" often refers to persons of rank in one's own firm and to high government officials.*

**DON'T**    capitalize the names of medical or surgical specialties
or the names of the specialists.

The internist referred him to a thoracic surgeon.

He is studying to be an emergency room specialist.

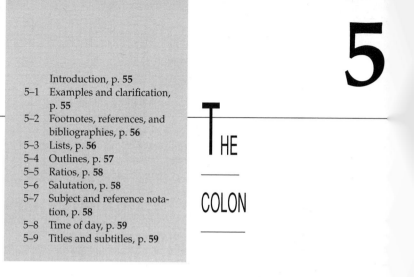

5

# 5

# THE

# COLON

## INTRODUCTION

Think of the colon as a pointer, drawing your attention to an important and concluding part. It is a mark of **anticipation.** It helps to couple separate elements that must be tied together but emphasized individually. Often the material to the right of the colon means the same as the material to the left of the colon.

## 5—1  EXAMPLES AND CLARIFICATION

**_DO_**     use a colon followed by a double space to introduce an example or to clarify an idea.

> **NOTE.**  *These ideas or examples are often introduced by the expressions* thus *or* that is; *or the expression could be supplied mentally.*

I see only one alternative:    chemotherapy.

You have only one goal here:    accuracy.

# 5 THE COLON

Notice please:  There will be no further parking allowed in the staff lot without a valid parking sticker.

Please place the following warning on the door to Room 16:  "Caution:  Radioactive materials in use."

There is one major problem with surgery in this young man:  his fear of being anesthetized.

## 5—2   FOOTNOTES, REFERENCES, AND BIBLIOGRAPHIES

**_DO_**   use a colon and double spacing between the title and subtitle and between the place of publication and the name of the publisher. Use a colon and no extra space between the volume number and page number. Use a period and double spacing between the name of the author and title and between the title and publication data.

Dorland's Illustrated Medical Dictionary, 27th ed. Philadelphia: WB Saunders Company; 1988.

CBE Style Manual Committee. CBE Style Manual: A Guide for Authors, Editors, and Publishers in the Biological Sciences, 5th ed. Bethesda, Maryland: Council of Biology Editors; 1983:50–53.

Esmann V, Geil JP, Droon S, et al. Prednisolone does not prevent post-herpetic neuralgia. Lancet Jul 1987; II:126–9.

## 5—3   LISTS

**_DO_**   use a colon followed by a double space to introduce a **list** preceded by a **complete sentence**. These lists are often introduced by the following expressed or implied words: _as follows, such as, namely, the following._

Please bring the following items with you to the hospital:   robe, slippers, toilet articles, and two pairs of pajamas.

The patient was treated for the following problems: insomnia, malaise, depression.

**DON'T** use a colon when the items of the list come immediately after a verb or preposition or after the words *because* or *that*.

The patient had:   a history of chronic obstructive lung disease and congestive heart failure. (**Incorrect**. Notice that this list is not introduced by a complete sentence; furthermore, the colon follows a verb.)

The patient had a history of chronic obstructive lung disease and congestive heart failure. (**Correct**)

**DON'T** use a colon when the sentence is continuous without it.

## 5—4   OUTLINES

*DO* use a colon followed by a double space after the introductory word or words in an outline, after the introductory word or words in a written history and physical, or in listing the patient's vital signs.

CHIEF COMPLAINT:   Hyperemesis.
PAST HISTORY:   Usual childhood diseases; no sequelae.
ALLERGY:   Patient denies any drug or food sensitivity.
VITAL SIGNS:   Temperature 101°. Pulse 58. BP 130/90.

# 5 THE COLON

**NOTE.** *The material after the colon in the previous examples begins with a capital letter.*

## 5—5 RATIOS

**_DO_** use a colon with no space on either side to express ratios. The colon takes the place of the word *to*.

The solution was diluted 1:100.
We had a 2:1 mix.

## 5—6 SALUTATION

**_DO_** place a colon after the salutation in a business letter when "mixed" punctuation is used.

**_OPTIONAL._** *When the salutation is informal and persons are addressed by their first names, you may use a comma.*

To Whom It May Concern:
Gentlemen:
Dear Dr. Berry:
Dear Bill: *or* Dear Bill,

## 5—7 SUBJECT AND REFERENCE NOTATION

**_DO_** use a colon and a double space to separate the reference or subject notation in the body of a letter.

RE:   Mary Ellen Wood

Re:   Mary Ellen Wood

Subject:   Soft-diet menus

## 5—8   TIME OF DAY

See also Rule 22–27.

***DO***   place a colon with no space on either side between the hours and minutes indicating the time of day in figures.

Her appointment is for 10:30 a.m.

**DON'T**   use a colon in expressions of military time.

She had an appointment at 1200 hours.
Patient was admitted at 1430.

## 5—9   TITLES AND SUBTITLES

***DO***   use a colon followed by a double space to separate titles from subtitles.

Medical Typing and Transcribing:   Techniques and Procedures

Chapter 1:   Your career as a transcriptionist

# 6

# THE

## COMMA

---

## INTRODUCTION

**_DO_**        use commas appropriately and sparingly.

**_DO_**        be able to justify your use of a comma or don't use it.

**DON'T**    create a comma fault: using only one of a pair of
             commas or using a comma to do the work of a semi-
             colon or colon.

**_DO_**        remember that commas are placed **inside** quotation
             marks and **outside** parentheses.

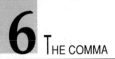

# 6 THE COMMA

## 6—1    ABBREVIATIONS

***DO***   use a comma or pair of commas to set off degrees and titles following a person's name.

John A. Meadows, M.D., saw the patient in consultation.

Mail this to John Vogt, Esq.

Nancy Casales, CMT, is the new president of the Mountain Meadows Chapter of AAMT.

***NOTE.*** *There is a trend to eliminate commas, particularly when meaning is not sacrificed. Some writers are not using commas to separate degrees and titles following a person's name. As always, follow the wishes of the bearer of the name.*

**DON'T**   place a comma before roman numerals indicating first, second, third, etc. or Jr. or Sr. following a name unless the bearer of the name prefers that usage.

Howard J. Matlock III

Carl A. Nichols Jr. was admitted to Ward B.

A Billroth I anastomosis was performed.

***DO***   use commas to separate abbrevations following a person's name. Place abbreviations in order of increasing distinction.

Neal J. Kaufman, M.D., FACCP
Rachel L. Connors Jr., M.D., L.L.B.

**DON'T** use a comma or pair of commas to set off *Inc.* and *Ltd.* following the name of a company *unless the firm follows that practice.*

He was covered by Bowen Myers Insurance Ltd.

I was employed by Peach Valley Medical Group Inc. for three years.

**_DO_** separate the parts of a name with a comma or commas when it is given in inverted order.

Jacobs, Barney K.
Kaufman, Neal J., M.D., FACP

**_DO_** use a comma or a pair of commas to set off the Latin abbreviations (e.g., i.e., viz.) and the spelled-out English versions (for example, that is, namely) when used at the end of a series or as a parenthetical expression. (See also Rule 1–11 concerning Latin abbreviations.)

He was allergic to most pet dander, e.g., that of dogs, cats, and rabbits.

## 6—2    ADDRESSES

See also Rule 6–18, *Place Names.*

**_DO_** use a comma to separate two different parts of a street address.

1335 11th Street, Apartment 3B

**_DO_**      use commas to separate all the elements of a complete
address.

Please mail this to my home address: 132 Winston
Street, Park Village, IL 60612.

## 6—3   APPOSITIVES

An appositive is a noun or pronoun that renames the noun or
pronoun that precedes it.

**_DO_**      separate nonessential appositives from the rest of the
sentence with a pair of commas.

John Munor, _your patient_, was admitted to Centre City
Hospital today.

Laralyn Abbott, _the head nurse_, summoned me to the
phone.

**DON'T**   separate an essential appositive in error. It is essential
if you need to know **which one**.

Your patient, _Ralph Swansdown_, died at 3:45 a.m.
(Incorrect. You need to know which patient.)

Your patient _Ralph Swansdown_ died at 3:45 a.m.
(Correct)

**OPTIONAL.**   _It is not necessary to put commas around
one-word appositives._

I myself will stay late and finish the report.

My cousin Pat just arrived in Spring Valley.

## 6—4   CLARITY

**_DO_**   use a comma or a pair of commas to facilitate reading the sentence or to indicate a required pause.

As demonstrated earlier, chemotherapy had little effect on the rate of tumor growth.

In 1990, 461 cases were reviewed by the Tumor Board.

Soon after, he got up and discharged himself from the hospital.

Dr. Powell, not Dr. Franklyn, delivered the infant.

She has bilateral tibial bowing, greater on the left than on the right.

After three, surgeries are not scheduled.

Subcutaneous tissue was closed using interrupted #4-0 Dexon, skin with the same material.

I would like her to be, and she probably will be, a candidate for heart surgery.

She required trifocal, not bifocal, lenses at this time.

**_DO_**   use a comma to separate repeated adjectives and adverbs.

He was very, very anxious to avoid any potentially claustrophobic encounters.

**_NOTE._**   _Not used for past perfect verb form._

He had had an automobile accident the previous week.

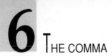

# 6 THE COMMA

## 6—5    COMPLIMENTARY CLOSE

**_DO_**    use a comma after the complimentary close when "mixed" punctuation is used in a letter.

Sincerely yours,

## 6—6    COMPOUND SENTENCE

See Rule 6–13, *Independent Clause*.

## 6—7    CONJUNCTIONS

See Rule 6–13, *Independent Clause*.

## 6—8    COORDINATE WORDS

See also Rule 6–19, *Series of Words*.

**_DO_**    use a comma when two consecutive adjectives independently modify the same noun. Separate them with a comma if a mental *and* can be placed between them or if the order in which they are used can be reversed.

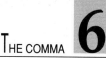

She is a spastic, retarded child.

It was a wide, deep wound.

He was left with windblown, contracted lips.

**DON'T** use a comma when the first adjective modifies the next adjective-noun combination.

She is an efficient, medical secretary. (incorrect)

He had crystal, clear urine. (incorrect)

## 6—9 DATES

*DO* use a comma to set off a year date that is used to explain a preceding date of the month.

He was born on March 3, 1933, in Reading, Pennsylvania.

Make her an appointment for Wednesday, July 6, 19XX.

**DON'T** use a comma when the complete date is not given.

He had surgery in April 1987 in Arizona.

She is to be seen again on February 3 at 10:30.

*DO* use a comma to separate the parts of a date in the date line of a letter.

November 11, 1989

# 6 The Comma

**DON'T** use a comma with the military date sequence.

11 November 1989

## 6—10    DIAGNOSIS

***DO*** use a comma to separate the parts of an inverted diagnosis. The correct inversion consists of what the problem is (comma) followed by where it is.

Atelectasis, left lower lobe.

Cataract, right eye.

Open fracture, tibiofibular, left lower extremity.

Serous otitis media, bilateral.

## 6—11    DIRECT ADDRESS

***DO*** use a comma or pair of commas to enclose a name used in direct address.

My thanks, Paul, for sending Mr. Byron in for consultation.

## 6—12    ESSENTIAL AND NONESSENTIAL WORDS, PHRASES, EXPRESSIONS, AND CLAUSES

Nonessential or nonrestrictive descriptive phrases or clauses add information that is **not** essential to the meaning of the sentence.

***DO***    use a comma or pair of commas to set off **nonessential** words, phrases, or clauses from the rest of the sentence.

Please notice, for example, the depth of the incision.

She should have, in my opinion, immediate surgery.

Paul Barth, who had surgery last month, came in for his final examination today.

He recovered well after his surgery, except for one episode of postsurgical hemorrhage.

The amniotic fluid had become brownish-green in color, suggesting some degree of fetal distress.

He is an excellent surgeon, whether or not you care for my opinion, and I feel that you must trust his judgment.

I would like her to be, and she probably will be, a candidate for heart surgery.

She required trifocal, not bifocal, lenses at this time.

Dr. Mitchell, having been in surgery since two this morning, collapsed on the day bed.

**DON'T** enclose essential material within commas. (This essential material will indicate who, what, why, when, or where.)

I want to examine all of the children, **when they have been prepared**. (incorrect)

Medical staff members, **who fail to attend the meeting**, will lose their consulting privileges. (incorrect)

Your patient, **Ethel Clifford**, saw me in consultation. (incorrect)

**DON'T** create a comma fault by leaving out one of the commas when a pair is required.

Her temperature, **which has been high** fell suddenly. (incorrect)

**DON'T** create a comma fault by inserting a comma where none belongs.

He had, had an automobile accident the previous week. (incorrect)

## 6—13  INDEPENDENT CLAUSE

**_DO_** use a comma to separate two or more independent clauses when they are joined by the conjunctions *and, or, nor, but, for, yet,* or *so.*

The diagnosis of urinary tract infection was made, and he was treated with Septra.

There is a story of a mild head injury at age ten, and apparently she was in a moderately severe motorcycle accident about fifteen years ago which resulted in a broken mandible.

The condition is now stationary and permanent, and he should be able to resume his normal work load.

Your appendix appears to be inflamed, but I do not believe that you need surgery at this time.

Your appendix appears to be inflamed, but not acutely. (Incorrect. The second phrase is dependent and must not be separated with a comma.)

*OPTIONAL.   Many modern writers are no longer using this comma. You may ask the author of your documents for his/her desires concerning this.*

**DON'T**  take this option when it makes the initial impression unclear.

I kicked the ball, and John accidentally slipped reaching for it. (A comma is needed in this sentence, or it might appear that you also kicked John when kicking the ball!)

**DON'T**  separate the parts of a compound from the main clause with a comma simply because a familiar conjunction is used.

Your appendix appears to be inflamed, but not acutely. (incorrect)

The child weighed 7 pounds at birth, and was the result of an uncomplicated pregnancy and delivery. (incorrect)

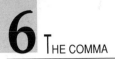

# 6 THE COMMA

You will recall that this introductory element can be thought of as being out of place in the sentence rather than at the end of a sentence in simple sentence order. Many of these introductory dependent phrases or clauses begin with words such as *since, because, after, about, during, by, if, when, while, although, unless, between, until, whenever, as,* and *before,* and with verb forms such as *hoping, believing, allowing, helping,* and *working.*

**_DO_**    use a comma to set off an introductory dependent phrase or clause.

After you have an x-ray, I will examine you. (simple introductory clause)

Dr. Chriswell was having difficulty dictating; however, after the equipment was adjusted, she was able to finish her reports. (part of the second independent clause)

Fully aware of his budget restrictions and with concern for the high cost of the equipment, Dr. Jellison approved the purchase of the word processor. (compound introductory phrase)

**DON'T**    separate the subject from the rest of the sentence in error.

To transcribe this accurately the first time, is the main goal. (not an introductory phrase — incorrect use of the comma)

**_DO_**    omit the comma after a brief (less than five words) introductory element if clarity is not sacrificed.

In the meantime he was discharged to his home.

If possible schedule the thoracotomy to follow the bronchoscopy.

## 6—15  NAMES

***DO***　　use commas to separate the first name from the last name when they are expressed in reverse order.

RE:　Lombardo, Vito

Falsworth, Marianne P. (Mrs. John R.)

## 6—16  NUMBERS

See Rule 6–9 for numbers in dates.

***DO***　　use commas to group numbers in units of three.

platelets 250,000; wbc 15,000

**DON'T**　use commas in four-digit numbers, street numbers, dates, ZIP codes, and some ID and technical numbers.

My bill to Medicare was $1250.

**DON'T**　use commas with the metric system or with decimals.

1 000 ml (correct) 1,000 ml (incorrect)

**DON'T** use commas to separate two units of the same dimension

The patient's height is 6 ft 3 in.

The infant was 3 days 4 hours old.

The surgery was completed in 2 hours 40 minutes.

She was a Gravida III Para II white female.*

*\*NOTE. Often expressed with lower case letters and arabic numerals. (See Chapter 22, Rule 22–21, Roman Numerals.)*

She was a gravida 3 para 2 white female.

## 6—17 PARENTHETICAL EXPRESSIONS

**_DO_** use a comma or a pair of commas to set off a parenthetical expression from the rest of the sentence. These expressions may begin, interrupt, or end a sentence and are always nonessential. (See also Rule 6–12, *Essential and Nonessential Words*.)

She said, *if my memory serves me right*, that she had graduated from medical school in 1987.

This burn needs immediate attention, *in my opinion*.

**_DO_** use a comma to set off a one-word parenthetical expression if you wish to indicate a pause.

*Furthermore*, she was to be seen by Dr. Sumners in surgical consultation.

He was *indeed* concerned about her progress. (Comma not needed for pause or emphasis here.)

**DON'T** use a comma to separate a parenthetical expression used as an adverb.

*However* sick he may be, it is not wise to intubate him at this time.

**NOTE.** *Following are some commonly used parenthetical expressions:* as already stated, in my opinion, as you probably know, without a doubt, nevertheless, as a matter of fact, between you and me, consequently, in the meantime, needless to say, therefore, by the way, for example.

## 6—18   PLACE NAMES

*DO* use a comma to set off the name of the state when the city precedes it.

The pacemaker was shipped to you from Syracuse, New York, by air express.

**DON'T** place a comma between the state name and the ZIP code. The ZIP code is considered part of the state name.

His address is 721 Thunderbird Drive, Tucson, Arizona 85719.

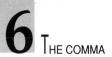

# 6 THE COMMA

## 6—19 SERIES OF WORDS, TESTS, STUDIES, VITALS, VALUES, AND SO FORTH

**_DO_** use a comma after each element or each pair of elements in a series of coordinate nouns, adjectives, verbs, or adverbs.

Please make a copy of the patient's operative report, pathology report, and consultation report for Dr. Reilly.

There were papers to be filed, charts to be sorted, ledgers to be posted.

**DON'T** use a comma between the last adjective and the word series it modifies.

The patient is a well-developed, well-nourished, elderly, white female telephone operator.

*OPTIONAL.   You may omit the comma before the conjunction if clarity is not sacrificed. Furthermore, no comma is used before the ampersand (&).*

*NOTE.   The option is **not** to be taken in this example because the color scheme would be unclear:*

The various hospital departments were decorated in green and yellow, blue and brown, and green and white.

**_DO_** use commas to separate abbreviations following a person's name, and place abbreviations in order of increasing distinction.

Neal J. Kaufman, M.D., FACCP
Rachel L. Connors Jr., M.D., L.L.B.

**_DO_**   use commas to separate groups of tests, studies, values, laboratory data, and so forth.

Speech, gag, jaw jerk, corneals, facial sensation are all intact.

Weight 83.5 kg, height 166 cm, temperature 98°, pulse 80/minute, respirations 20/minute, blood pressure 120/86.

**DON'T**   use commas to separate more complex value groups. (See Chapter 32, _Semicolon_ and Chapter 5, _Colon_.)

Blood pressure 194/97; pulse 127; respirations 32, regular, and gasping.

_and also correct:_

Blood pressure: 194/97; pulse: 127;
respirations: 32, regular, and gasping.

**DON'T**   use commas to separate two units of the same dimension.

The patient's height was 6 ft 3 in.

The infant was 3 days 4 hours old.

The surgery was completed in 2 hours 40 minutes.

She was a Gravida III Para II white female.

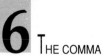

**DON'T** separate sets of words incorrectly.

There was no change in the cervix with that structure continuing to be long closed, and posterior (Incorrect: A comma is required after *long*, since the cervix is not *long closed* but long and closed.)

There were normal reflexes of suck, root, and startle. (correct separation)

Serum electrolytes, alkaline phosphatase, BUN, creatinine, glucose, and calcium will be checked. (correct)

**_DO_** use commas to separate a series of short independent clauses. (See Chapter 32, *Semicolon*, concerning the usual punctuation used to separate a series of independent clauses.)

She was upset about being seen, she resented my intrusion, and she said so.

# 7

# COMPOUNDS

## INTRODUCTION

Compounds consist of two or more separate words and/or phrases that are used as a single word, often with the help of a hyphen to join them. It is often difficult to know if a set of words should be typed as one word, two or more separate words, or as a compound hyphenated word. Often there are no specific rules to follow for these compound words. (Consider *chin bone* and *cheekbone*.) These general rules will assist you with most words. Since this is also a spelling problem, consult the dictionary for specific compound help. (See Rules 31–23 and 31–24 for spelling reference books.) (See also Chapter 15, *Hyphen Use and Word Division*.)

# 7 COMPOUNDS

## 7—1    CHEMICAL COMPOUNDS

**_DO_**    join prefixed locants (the chemical location in the molecule) and descriptors to the name of the organic compound with a hyphen.

    beta-sitosterol        cis-dichloroethene
    2-hexanone

**_DO_**    use a hyphen to separate the abbreviations for known amino acid sequences.

    Lys-Asp-Gly

    **NOTE.**    *Unknown sequences are enclosed in parentheses and separated by commas.*

**_DO_**    join chemical compounds and formulas with hyphens and closeup punctuation.

9-nitroanthra(1,9,4,10)bis(1)oxathiazone-2,7-bisdioxide

## 7—2    COINED COMPOUNDS

**_DO_**    join a single letter to a word to form a coined compound.

    x-ray        Z-plasty        S-shaped
    T-cell        U-bag           X-Acto
    X-rated      T-wave        V-neck

**_DO_**    join a number to a word to form a coined compound phrase.

    SMA-l         alpha-l        profile-1

## 7—3    COMPOUND MODIFIER BEFORE A NOUN

**_DO_**    use a hyphen to join two or more words that have the force of a single modifier before a noun.

figure-of-eight sutures
self-addressed envelope
low-grade fever
self-inflicted knife wound
two-pack-a-day smoker
happy-go-lucky personality
well-known speaker
mouth-to-mouth resuscitation
through-and-through sutures
ill-defined tumor mass
up-to-date report
large-for-date fetus
non-English-speaking patient
diagnosis-related groups

She is a well-developed, well-nourished, 35-year-old black female.

She was seen today in final follow-up examination.

An end-to-end anastomosis was performed.

The resident consulted the alcoholism counselors on his two MAST-positive patients.

This is a very up-to-date reference for drug names.

**DON'T**    use a hyphen when the compound follows the noun.

I want these records brought **up to date**.

She appears to be **well nourished**.

**DON'T**   make a compound modifier with an adverb ending in *ly*.

That was a poorly dictated report.

She is a moderately obese waitress.

*DO*   make sure that a compound is intended.

We applied a long-leg cast.
(The cast is for a long leg.)

We applied a long leg cast.
(The cast for the leg is long.)

There was a soft-tissue lesion on the surface.
(The lesion is composed of soft tissue.)

There was a soft tissue lesion.
(The lesion is soft.)

*DO*   use a hyphen to join two or more words used to describe a noun when clarity is required.

brown-bag lunch

small-town physician

long-awaited diagnosis

*DO*   hyphenate modifiers with a capitalized second element.

pro-American advertising
anti-Asian outburst
pre-Elizabethan period
non-English speaking

## 7—4 COORDINATE EXPRESSIONS AFTER THE VERB

See also Rule 7–11.

**_DO_**   use a hyphen to join coordinate expressions after the verb.

The waiting room was painted a sort of yellow-orange.

That remark was well-taken.

The patient's expression was happy-sad.

That income was tax-exempt.

The old gentleman was stone-deaf.

## 7—5 LATIN COMPOUNDS

**DON'T**   use hyphens with Latin compounds such as _ad hoc, bona fide, prima facie, per capita._

I appointed an _ad hoc_ committee to study that.

Carcinoma was found _in situ._

She was part of the _in vivo_ fertility program.

# 7 COMPOUNDS

**_DO_**    use a hyphen to join compound nouns, compound surnames, and compound eponyms.

A Davis-Crowe mouth gag was used.

She is of Mexican-American ancestry.

Mary Smyth-Reynolds was in today for her annual Pap smear.

Antonio is the new secretary-treasurer.

Dr. Asser is Cedar's chief-of-staff.

He is doing research with the Epstein-Barr virus.

**DON'T**    hyphenate names that are unhyphenated names of a single person.

Austin Moore hip prosthesis **not** Austin-Moore

_**NOTE.** There is no hyphen between the words_ Austin _and_ Moore _because the prosthesis was invented by Dr. Thomas Austin Moore and not, as one might think, by two persons respectively surnamed Austin and Moore. (Check your references when you are not sure.)_

## 7—7 NUMBERS AND FRACTIONS COMPOUNDED WITH WORDS

**_DO_**    use a hyphen when numbers are compounded with words and they have the force of a single modifier.

one-third share

four-fifths majority

35-hour week

2-inch incision

Four-vessel angiography showed a narrowing of the left carotid artery.

**EXCEPTION.**  *There is only a 3 percent difference.*

**DON'T**  use a hyphen when the compound follows the noun.

He is a 56-year-old janitor in no acute distress.

The janitor is 56 years old.

## 7—8   NUMBERS, COMPOUND AND MULTIPLE

***DO***  use a hyphen to separate compound written-out numbers between 21 and 99 and written-out simple fractions.

Fifty-five medical transcriptionists attended the meeting last night.

Ninety-nine percent of the time I am confident of the diagnosis.

Paresis was noted in one-half of her left thumb.

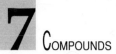

# 7 COMPOUNDS

**_DO_**    use the hyphen to attach the number modifier to the noun when the number is preceded by another number.

inserted two 8-inch drains
ordered six 2-gauge needles

## 7—9    PLURAL FORMATION OF COMPOUNDS

**_DO_**    add the appropriate plural ending to compound nouns written as one word.

fingerbreadths        teaspoonfuls        spokesmen

**_DO_**    add the appropriate plural ending to the word that is the essential noun in compound nouns written with hyphens or spaces.

sisters-in-law        surgeons general
chiefs-of-staff

## 7—10    PREFIX COMPOUNDED COMMON NOUNS AND ADJECTIVES

**_DO_**    use a hyphen with compound words beginning with _ex, self,_ and _vice_; also join various other prefixes to avoid an awkward combinations of letters, such as two or three identical vowels in a sequence.

self-inflicted wound        ex-patient
intra-arterial pressure     micro-organism

**DON'T** use a hyphen with the compound words beginning with the prefixes *ante, anti, co, contra, counter, de, inter, intra, multi, non, out, over, post, pre, pro, pseudo, re, semi, trans, un, sub, supra,* and *under* unless the word has identical letters in a sequence.

| | | |
|---|---|---|
| retype | anti-inflammatory | undernourished |
| preoperative | postoperative | pre-evaluation |
| antenatal | post-traumatic | antidepressant |
| semiprone | nondrinker | outpatient |
| ante mortem | anti-immune | postmortem |
| intra-abdominal | | |

*EXCEPTIONS:*

**No Hyphen:**

| | |
|---|---|
| transsacral | preempt |
| preeclampsia | preemployment |
| reexamine | reenter |
| reemploy | |

**With Hyphen:**
pre-position (to position again)
re-form (to form again)
re-mark (to mark again)
re-treat (to treat again)
re-creation (to create again)
re-infuse (to infuse again)
non-Hodgkins (See Rule 7–11.)

**DO** use a hyphen with compound words beginning with the prefix *extra* when the meaning is *additonal* or the word root begins with an *a*.

extra-large          extra-apical

**DON'T** use a hyphen with compound words beginning with the prefix *extra* when the meaning is *outside of.*

extradural          extrathoracic
extracurricular

## 7—11    PREFIX COMPOUNDED PROPER NOUNS

**_DO_**   use a hyphen to join a prefix to the proper noun in a compound.

> un-American
> pseudo-Christian
> non-Hodgkins

> The estimated date of confinement is sometime in mid-May.

## 7—12    "STATUS POST"

**DON'T**   hyphenate the phrase "status post."

> status postoperative
> status post knee joint prosthesis

**DON'T**   join "status post" to the word that follows it.

> status post hernia repair
> status post vascular shunt

## 7—13    SUFFIX COMPOUNDS

**_DO_**   use hyphens to form compounds with the suffixes _-elect, -designate, -odd,_ and _-in._

> president-elect
> thirty-odd minutes
> shoo-in
> ambassador-designate

**_DO_**   use a hyphen when a compound consists of an adjective plus a noun plus *-ed*. This combination is used both before and after the noun.

She was a good-natured patient.
The patient was good-natured.

The middle-aged man was interviewed.
The man we interviewed was middle-aged.

I removed a small-sized tumor.
The tumor was small-sized.

There was a short-lived break in the schedule.
The break was short-lived.

## 7—14   SUSPENDING HYPHEN

**_DO_**   use a suspending hyphen to connect a series of compound modifiers.

There were small- and large-sized cysts scattered throughout the parenchyma.

He has a two- or three-month convalescence ahead of him.

She had first- and second-degree burns on her upper extremities.

# 8

# Dash

## INTRODUCTION

A dash is made on the keyboard with two hyphens. There is no space before, between, or after the two hyphens.

**_DO_**  use the dash *very* sparingly; with overuse, it loses its effect.

**DON'T**  use a dash when another punctuation mark will do.

## 8—1  AMPLIFY OR EXPLAIN

**_DO_**  use a single dash to emphasize, amplify, explain, or summarize a statement.

As I told you before, she is scheduled for internal mammary artery implantation — not femoral artery implantation.

The diagnosis is grim — I feel helpless.

# 8 DASH

## 8—2 INTERRUPTION

**_DO_**   use a pair of dashes for a forceful break or interruption.

I want you to — no, I insist that you — consult a surgeon about the growth in your breast.

## 8—3 OMISSION

**_DO_**   use a single dash to indicate the omission of letters or words.

His not showing up on time for surgery put us in one h— of a bind.

**DON'T**   use the dash to indicate an omission when you simply have nothing particular in mind to say.

## 8—4 PARENTHETICAL EXPRESSION

**_DO_**   use the dash instead of commas when commas have been used to punctuate the expression itself.

The entire x-ray department — physicians, technicians, therapists, transcriptionists, secretaries, clerks — was completely engrossed in the demonstration of the new equipment.

## 8—6    SUMMARY

___DO___    use a single dash for summary.

Pediatrics, obstetrics, psychiatry — these were my
favorite rotations.

**9**

# Drugs

## AND

## DRUG

## REFERENCES

## 9—1    ABBREVIATIONS

**_DO_**    avoid typing an abbreviation if it can be misread and/or misinterpreted in a chart note.

DC can be translated as *discharge* or *discontinue*, thus a patient could be sent home too early or taken off medication too soon.

DPT stands for two different injectables — a painkiller/tranquilizer combination (Demerol, Phenergan, and Thorazine) or an immunization (diphtheria/pertussis/tetanus).

DW indicates dextrose (sugar) in water, distilled water, or deionized water.

OD for *once daily* can also be translated to mean *right eye (oculus dexter), overdose, on duty,* or *doctor of optometry.*

ON can be misread as the word *on, overnight, Ortho-Novum* (birth control pills), or *every night.*

## 9—2   BRAND NAME

**_DO_**     capitalize the first letter of the proprietary or trade name of a drug that is copyrighted by the manufacturer.

| **Brand** | **Generic** |
|-----------|-------------|
| Scotch tape | cellophane tape |
| Miltown tablets | meprobamate |
| Demerol | meperidine |

**EXCEPTION.**   *Maintain any idiosyncratic capitalization used by the proprietor of the brand name.*

NegGram   pHisoHex   GoLYTELY   HydroDIURIL

**DON'T**   use lower case after a hyphen

Ser-Ap-Es

## 9—3   CHEMICAL NAME

**_DO_**     begin the chemical name of a drug in lower case, in-serting commas and hyphens as the formula warrants.

2-methyl-2-n-propyl-1-1,3-propanediol dicarbamate

## 9—4   CHEMOTHERAPEUTIC DRUGS

**DO**    use acronyms when a patient receives combination chemotherapeutic agents for treatment.

**B-DOPA** for bleomycin, DTIC, Oncovin, prednisone, Adriamycin

**5-FU** for 5-fluorouracil

## 9—5   DESIGNER DRUGS

**DO**    type acronyms or slang names when a physician dictates such in reference to designer drugs in medical reports.

MPPP   MDMA called *Ecstasy* or *Adam*   PEPAP PCP   or *Angel Dust*   heroin or *China White*

## 9—6   DOSAGE

**DO**    be careful in transcribing drug dosages. Incorrect numbers could mean a fatal error.

If Q.D. is mistaken for O.D., medication meant to be given once a day could be applied to the right eye.

If U for units is mistaken for a 0 (zero), the dosage will be multiplied ten times. (Spell out *units*.)

# 9 DRUGS AND DRUG REFERENCES

## 9—7 EXPERIMENTAL DRUGS

**_DO_**    use the manufacturer's code number to identify an experimental unapproved drug not yet assigned a USAN name.

PAA-3854

## 9—8 GENERIC NAME

**_DO_**    type or use lower case letters to spell nonproprietary or generic names (some examples given are not drugs).

| Generic | Brand |
|---|---|
| cellophane tape | Scotch tape |
| meprobamate | Miltown tablets |

**DON'T**    use the lower case if the generic and brand names sound alike.

Adrenalin          adrenaline

**_DO_**    be consistent in choosing to use upper- or lower-case letters. Some drug names have identical brand name and generic name spelling.

He is on Dilantin, SSKI drops, Choledyl, and Prednisone. (*Prednisone* can be generic or brand. Since the other drugs referred to are brand name drugs, it can be assumed that this drug is being referred to, as well, by brand name.)

## 9—9    NUMBERS

**_DO_**    use figures in all expressions pertaining to drugs, including strength, dosage, and directions.

b.i.d., twice a day, or 2 times a day

q4h, q.4h., or every 4 hours

He is to take Tofranil, 75 mg/day x 3 days to be increased to 100-150 mg/day if there is no response.

The directions for her Motrin were 400 mg q4h PRN for pain.

One generally gives 6.2 mg/kg to 9.4 mg/kg for those children 9 years old or younger.

**_EXCEPTION:_**  *The number one (1) may be written out or expressed as a numeral. If it is followed by an abbreviated unit of measure, the numeral should be used.*

Triaminic 1 tsp. q4h

**_DO_**    for the sake of clarity, omit commas between drug names, dosages, and instructions.

The patient was given Pen-Vee K 500 mg q.i.d. for ten days.

**_NOTE._**  *Since this example shows a nonessential clause, it should have commas and may be seen with commas as a variable.*

The patient was given Pen-Vee K, 500 mg, q.i.d. for ten days.

**_DO_**   use a comma or semicolon when typing a series that includes drugs, dosages, and instructions.

The patient was sent home on Norpace 150 mg q6h; Procardia 20 mg q6h; and digoxin 0.125 mg q.a.m.

*or*

The patient was sent home on Surmontil 25 mg t.i.d., nitrogylcerin 0.4 mg sublingual p.r.n., and Benadryl 50 mg q6h p.r.n.


## 9—10    RADIOACTIVE DRUGS

**_DO_**   begin radioactive pharmaceuticals with a capital letter and use hyphens where indicated. It is optional to show super- or subscript.

I-131,  $^{131}$I,  Tc-99m,  T3  uptake,  $T_3$  uptake,  T4 (thyroxine),  $T_4$


## 9—11    REFERENCES

**_DO_**   carefully check any drug names in question for the correct spelling; and if still uncertain about what drug name was dictated, leave a space on the line and write a note to the dictator, describing how the drug name sounded. (See Chapter 31, *Reference Materials and Publications,* for a listing of pharmaceutical reference books.)

## 9—12    SOUND-ALIKE, LOOK-ALIKE DRUG NAMES

**_DO_**    flag a transcript if you are unable to decipher a physician's handwriting from the patient's record or are unable to understand the dictated sound-alike or look-alike drug.

| | |
|---|---|
| Bicillin | V-Cillin |
| Coumadin | coumarin |
| digoxin (pronounced di-JOX-in) | Desoxyn |

# 10

# $E$DITING

---

## INTRODUCTION

**_DO_**  transcribe exactly what is dictated, keeping the following rules or exceptions in mind. Far more editorial latitude is permitted in private medical offices and small hospital departments than in large institutions or transcription services.

## 10—1  ABBREVIATIONS

**_DO_**  spell out abbreviations in the diagnosis section of medical reports so there is no chance for misinterpretation. The diagnosis section may appear as an impression, pre- or postoperative diagnosis, discharge diagnosis, or differential diagnosis.

FINAL DIAGNOSIS: ASHD. (incorrect)
FINAL DIAGNOSIS: Arteriosclerotic heart disease. (correct)

IMPRESSION: CVA (incorrect)
IMPRESSION: Chronic villous arthritis (correct)

PREOPERATIVE DIAGNOSIS: DVIU (incorrect)
PREOPERATIVE DIAGNOSIS: Direct vision internal urethrotomy (correct)

DISCHARGE DIAGNOSIS: GVHD (incorrect)
DISCHARGE DIAGNOSIS: Graft-versus-host disease (correct)

DIFFERENTIAL DIAGNOSIS: VZV (incorrect)
DIFFERENTIAL DIAGNOSIS: Varicella zoster virus (correct)

## 10—2   ARTICLES

**_DO_**   insert or delete articles, such as *a, an, the*, to gramatically improve sentences when they have been added or inadvertently omitted from the dictation. This may occur when listening to a dictator who has a foreign accent.

Patient had colitis in past. (incorrect)
The patient had colitis in the past. (correct)

## 10—3   BRIEF FORMS

**_DO_**   spell out brief forms. However, when a brief form is dictated, it can be typed as a brief form unless it might be misread and/or misinterpreted in the report. Likewise, brief forms may be typed in chart notes unless they might be misread or misinterpreted.

Temp 101. (incorrect)
Temperature 101. (correct)

The sputum culture grew out H. flu. (incorrect)
The sputum culture grew out Hemophilus influenzae.
(correct)
The sputum culture grew out H. influenzae. (correct)

The patient had a right thoracotomy for removal of
cocci nodules. (incorrect)
The patient had a right thoracotomy for removal of
coccidioidomycosis nodules. (correct)

## 10—4    FLAGGING, CARDING, TAGGING, OR MARKING

**_DO_**      flag, card, tag, or mark if you cannot quite hear or
understand any word or phrase and leave a blank. Attach the note to the transcript with a brief description
of where the blank is located (Fig. 10–1).

The middlehear was hair contain' . . . (sounds like)
The middle ear was air containing . . . (actually dictated)

## 10—5    FOREIGN DICTATORS

### Articles

**_DO_**      insert or delete articles, such as *a, an, the*, to grammati-
cally improve sentences when they have been added
or inadvertently omitted from the dictation. This may
occur when listening to a dictator who has a foreign
accent. The word *the* frequently will sound like *de* or *ze*.

Patient had colitis in past. (incorrect)
The patient had colitis in the past. (correct)

Dear Doctor _____ :

RE: Patient name _____

Report name _____

Date dictated _____

☐ Please see blank on page ___ , paragraph _____ of this report. It sounded like _____

☐ Dictate more slowly and distinctly.

☐ Spell proper names.

☐ Spell unusual words in address.

☐ Spell patient names.

☐ Spell new and unusual surgical instruments.

☐ Spell new drug names.

☐ Spell new laboratory tests.

☐ Indicate unusual punctuation.

☐ Indicate closing salutation.

☐ Indicate your title.

☐ Indicate end of letter.

☐ Give dates of reports.

☐ Speak louder.

☐ Give patient's hospital number.

☐ Please read the area of this report indicated by the penciled checkmark for accuracy.

☐ Your dictation was cut off. Please fill in the rest of the report or redictate.

Thank you. Please return this note with corrections via hospital mail to:

Transcriptionist _____

Telephone No. _____ Date _____

**Figure 10–1.** An example of a flagging or tagging note to be appended to a medical transcript for solving problem dictation. This form may be printed on colored paper.

## English Sound Substitutes

Foreign dictators may substitute certain letter sounds in error and this misleads the typist in spelling the word correctly. Some of these problem English sound substitutes are as follows:

A dictator unable to dictate the TH sound may substitute S for TH.
*sink* for *think*

The G sound may be replaced by the K sound.
*tinkling* for *tingling*

An R may be substituted for L.
*plesent* for *present*

An L may be substituted for R.
*lelief* for *relief*

A V may be pronounced as B.
*bery* for *very*

A short i sound may be pronounced as a long e.
*deestress* for *distress*

A long a sound is frequently pronounced as AH.
*vahgus* nerve for *vagus* nerve

## Grammar

Frequently correction of grammar is necessary but should be edited only to the extent that it does not change the meaning of the dictation. Sentence structure may need rearrangement. Remember medical language may not be changed without permission from the physician/dictator.

## Punctuation

A foreign dictator may pronounce the punctuation mark *comma* (,) as koma, and the student may think of the medical term coma, which is incorrect.

Some dictators from a foreign country denote *period* (.) by saying *full stop*.

## Word Beginnings

Foreign dictators sound word beginnings quite differently than an English speaking dictator. Some of these problem word beginnings are as follows:

An H may be substituted for F.
*hefty-six* for *fifty-six*

Some dictators use the K sound for words beginning with C that in English are sounded as S.
*kefalus* for *cephalus*

Dictators with Hispanic heritage may pronounce an X as S.
*espire* for *expire*
*estend* for *extend*
*eshale* for *exhale*

Dictators with Hispanic heritage may add an EH sound before words that begin with S.
*eskin* for *skin*
*espine* for *spine*
*estone* for *stone*

## Word Endings

**_DO_**  insert or delete word endings if sounds have been added or endings have been inadvertently omitted from the dictation (e.g., *chesteh* for *chest*). Some problem endings for foreign dictators are as follows:

*-ed* This ending is sometimes pronounced as a separate syllable
explain-*ed* for *explain*

*-s, -ed, -al, -ive* These endings may be dropped by the foreign dictator.

*-s* A word ending not used in English may be dictated.
*abdomens* for *abdomen*

*-d* The final d sound of a word is sometimes pronounced as a t.
*hat* for *had*

*-us* may be pronounced as *-oose*.
*vagoose* nerve for *vagus* nerve

## 10—6  GRAMMAR

See also Rule 10–13, *Verb-Subject Agreement*.

**_DO_**  change improper grammar. Make sure that the verb and noun match in number.

There was fifteen members present.   were (correct)

The adnexa was negative.   were (correct)

Then 5 ml of solution were injected into the intravenous fluid.   was (correct)

# 10 EDITING

**_DO_**   use proper parts of speech.

The patient was found laying on the floor. lying (correct)

**_DO_**   use proper words.

There was no reoccurrence of his tumor. recurrence (correct)

**_DO_**   use nouns and adjectives correctly.

He was scheduled for replacement of his aorta valve. aortic (correct)

**_DO_**   use proper singular or plural nouns.

The conjunctiva were bilaterally inflamed. conjunctivae (correct)

Pulse 72 and regular, respiration 18. respirations (correct)

**_DO_**   position the modifiers correctly.

The patient had a hysterectomy leaving one tube and ovary in Jacksonville. (incorrect)

The patient had a hysterectomy in Jacksonville, leaving one tube and ovary. (correct)

**_DO_**   use the **past tense** in the past history portion of a report, in the discharge summary, or to discuss an expired patient.

I saw your patient in the office yesterday. She is complaining of pain in the left lower quadrant of about a week's duration.
is complaining (incorrect)
*was* complaining (correct)

___
**_DO_** use **present tense** to discuss the current illness or disease in the history and physical.

___

10—7    INCONSISTENCIES AND REDUNDANCIES

___

**_DO_** delete redundancies and repair inconsistencies and inaccuracies.

The patient had no sisters and no siblings. (incorrect)
The patient has no siblings. (correct)

The suture was closed with #6-0 silk sutures. (incorrect)
The wound was closed with #6-0 silk sutures. (correct)

WBC was 10,000 with 7l segs, 2l% lymphs, and 8% monos. (incorrect)
WBC was 10,000 with 7l% segs, 2l% lymphs, and 8% monos. (correct)

Babinski negative (incorrect statement)
Babinski present or Babinski absent (correct statements)

*NOTE.  If you recognize an inconsistency or an inaccuracy but are not technically knowledgeable, ask for help.*

# 10 Editing

**_DO_**     double-check drug names or medical words when a dictator has carefully spelled them out if you have any doubt about their accuracy.

**_DO_**     determine what a foreign dictator intends to say and type it preserving the integrity of the meaning of the sentence if the dictator uses grammar rules governing his or her own language.

> The incision was prolonged. (incorrect)
> The incision was extended. (correct)

> The patient's painful feets had disappeared. (incorrect)
> The patient's foot pain had disappeared. (correct)

10—9    NORMAL AND NEGATIVE FINDINGS

**DON'T**    delete negative or normal findings.

10—10    ORGANIZATION AND WRITING STYLE

**_DO_**     adjust or rephrase, but preserve the exact meaning of the author or dictator.

> The patient drinks several beers per day, occasional cigars and cigarettes. (incorrect)

> The patient drinks several beers per day and occasionally smokes cigars and cigarettes. (correct)

## 10—11    PROOFREADING

See Chapter 28, *Proofreading and Revisions.*

## 10—12    SLANG, VULGAR, AND INFLAMMATORY REMARKS

Medical slang that is acceptable and commonly used by physicians is seen in Chapter 33, *Slang and Unusual Medical Terms.* Rules presented in this section refer to questionable slang.

***DO***       check with your supervisor before transcribing or editing questionable remarks.

          The patient was stupid, a crock (hypochondriac), and dumb.
The lousy surgeon used a quack treatment.
The nitwit charge nurse should have brought it to my attention.

***DO***       contact the dictator and diplomatically and tactfully question his or her use of the questionable words before they become a permanent part of the patient's medical record.

## 10—13    VERB-SUBJECT AGREEMENT

***DO***       correct verb-subject dictation errors. Remember the verb must agree in number with its subject.

          There appears to be old healed rib fractures of the ninth and tenth ribs. (incorrect)
There appear to be old healed rib fractures of the ninth and tenth ribs. (correct)

*RATIONALE.* *The subject is the word* fractures *and it must agree in number with the verb* appear.

No evidence of any overlapping sutures are seen. (incorrect)
No evidence of any overlapping sutures is seen. (correct)

*RATIONALE.* *The verb must agree in number with the subject of the sentence and not with an intervening prepositional phrase.*

No adenopathy, lumps, or masses is seen in the chest. (incorrect)
No adenopathy, lumps, or masses are seen in the chest. (correct)

*RATIONALE.* *When there is a series, the verb agrees in number with the nearest subject.*

Ultrasound and whirlpool therapy were used. (incorrect)
Ultrasound and whirlpool therapy was used. (correct)

*RATIONALE.* *The subject* therapy *is singular and, though modified by two adjectives, takes a singular verb.*

# 11

# Envelope

# PREPARATION

## 11—1    FOLDING AND INSERTING

See Chapter 17, *Letter Format.*

## 11—2    MAILING ADDRESS

***DO***     use the nine-digit ZIP code to expedite and reduce mailing costs when using bulk mail processing.

San Francisco, CA 94120-7168     Portland, Oregon 97204-2628
San Diego, CA 92109-3602     New York, New York 10005-4101

***DO***     use single spacing, and block each line at the left, giving the name of the person to whom you are writing, the street address (post office box number or rural route number), and city (written in full), state, and ZIP code. See example on next page.

Marvin O'Connor, M. D.
2458 West Main Street
Dayton, OH 45439-2017

**_DO_** put the apartment or suite number after the street address or on the line above.

Mrs. Arthur Gildea
1826 Lucretia Road, Apt. 3D
Oxnard, CA 93030-8213

*or*

Mrs. Arthur Gildea
Apartment 3D
1826 Lucretia Road
Oxnard, CA 93030-8213

**_DO_** capitalize the first letter of each word except prepositions, conjunctions, and articles used in a name or title. The United States Postal Service prefers all capital letters, but this is not required. Punctuation (periods with abbreviations and commas) is also not required. Optical character readers can read the traditional style of address as well as the all-cap style.

**traditional:**
James B. Peter, M. D.
4500 Oregon Street
Portland, OR 97204-2628

*or*

**optical character reader:**
JAMES B PETER MD
4500 OREGON STREET
PORTLAND OR 97204 2628

***DO***    give a two-letter abbreviation for the state name. (See Chapter 2, *Address Formats for Letters and Forms of Address*, and Chapter 42, *ZIP Codes*, Rule 42–9.) See Figure 1–1.

***DO***    leave 1 to 3 spaces between the state name and the ZIP Code.

***DO***    type an attention line (when one is necessary) on the second line below the inside address starting at the left margin or as the second line of the address.

**traditional:**
National Paper Company
Attention: Frank Honeywell
1492 Columbus Avenue, North
New York, NY 10005-4101

*or*

**optical character reader:**
NATIONAL PAPER CO
ATTN FRANK HONEYWELL
1492 COLUMBUS AVE N
NEW YORK NY 10005 4101

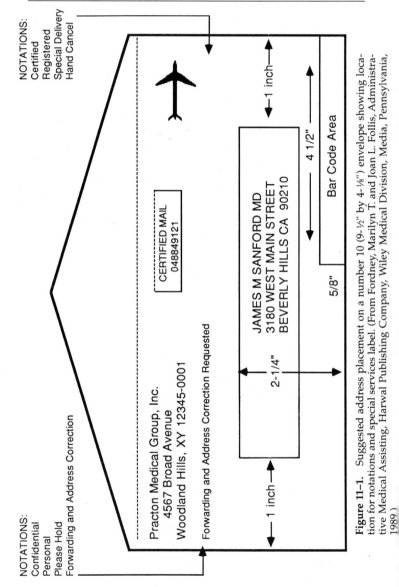

**Figure 11-1.** Suggested address placement on a number 10 (9-½" by 4-⅛") envelope showing location for notations and special services label. (From Fordney, Marilyn T. and Joan L. Follis, Administrative Medical Assisting, Harwal Publishing Company, Wiley Medical Division, Media, Pennsylvania, 1989.)

**DO**      use the name of the institution or company name as the first line if no person's name is available.

**DO**      type the address block for optical character reader processing no higher than 2-1/4 inches from the bottom edge of the envelope, no lower than 5/8 inch from the bottom edge, and no closer than 1 inch from either the left or the right edges of the envelope.

**DO**      use single spacing, abbreviations, all-caps, no punctuation, and block each line at the left, giving the name of the person to whom you are writing, the street address (post office box number or rural route number), and city, state, and ZIP code. Optical character readers can read traditional style of address as well as the all-cap style.

MARTIN J LEVINE MD
4900 ASCOT RD
HOUSTON TX 77042 1839

**DON'T**   use both post office box number and street address when both are known.

**DO**      Use the post office box number.

**DON'T**   allow any notations to fall alongside or below the area established for the mailing address, since this will interfere with OCR processing.

**DON'T**   use a script or italic typeface.

**DO**      use the foreign country's name on the last line in all capital letters.

## 11—4    PERSONAL NOTATIONS

***DO***    list personal notations (confidential, personal, please hold, forwarding and address correction requested) below the return name and address beginning on line 9 or on the third line below the return address. Begin each main word with a capital and align at the left with the return name and address.

## 11—5    POSTAL (MAILING) NOTATIONS

***DO***    list mailing notations (special delivery, registered, certified, hand cancel) in all-capital letters in the upper right corner of the envelope beginning on line 9 or on the third line below the bottom edge of the stamp. The notation should end about one-half inch (5 pica spaces, 6 elite spaces) from the right margin. Be sure to leave room for the postage.

## 11—6    RETURN ADDRESS

***DO***    list a return name and address in the upper left corner of the envelope beginning on line 3 about one-half inch (5 pica spaces, 6 elite spaces) in from the left edge.

## 11—7    ZIP CODE

See Chapter 42, *ZIP Codes*.

# 12

## Eponyms

## INTRODUCTION

Medical eponyms are adjectives used to describe specific treatments, operations, surgical instruments, diseases, parts of the anatomy, laboratory procedures, pharmacology, and microbiology. Each of these words is the surname (or an adjective formed from the surname) of an individual who is prominently connected with the development or discovery of the disease, instrument, surgical procedure, and so forth.

This is not a reference list of eponyms, but it is important that you have one. Always carefully check the spelling of these difficult terms by consulting a dictionary or other reference book. One should look for the eponym by checking under the noun that accompanies it; e.g., to find the correct spelling for *Abbe's anemia* look under the listing *anemia*.

See Chapter 3, *Apostrophe*, for proper punctuation of eponyms.

*NOTE.  It is important to note that more and more writers are making exceptions to the possessive rule by not showing the possessive with an eponym. One might expect a change in the rule with more eponyms treated as the eponyms for surgical instruments are treated. In checking dictionaries and other reference books, one finds conflicting spellings: one showing the eponym with the possessive and one showing it without.*

**DO**        capitalize all eponyms but **not** the nouns that accompany them.

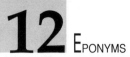 

## 12—1   ANATOMY

There are literally thousands of eponyms that refer to various parts of the human body. If generic terms are available to describe a body part or organ, they should be used in preference to the eponym.

**_DO_**    capitalize an eponym that refers to a part of the anatomy and show the possessive (*'s*) when appropriate to do so.

Bartholin's glands          Golgi complex
Beale's ganglion            Flack's node
Mauthner's membrane         circle of Willis
Purkinje's fibers           Stensen's duct
bundle of His               Broca's area
islands (or islets) of Langerhans

**DON'T**   capitalize most words **derived** from eponymic names.

fallopian tube              eustachian tube
malpighian bodies

## 12—2   DISEASES AND SYNDROMES

This is a list that is constantly growing as new diseases are identified and named or combinations of symptoms are grouped into a new syndrome. Some diseases have a common name, an eponymic description, and an abbreviation.

HW syndrome
*or*
Hayem-Widal syndrome
*or*
acquired hemolytic jaundice

HW disease
*or*
His-Werner disease
*or*
shinbone fever *or* five-day fever


SS
*or*
Strachan-Scott syndrome
*or*
avitaminosis $B_2$


**_DO_**  capitalize an eponym that refers to a disease, condition, reflex, phenomenon, or syndrome and show the possessive (*'s*) when appropriate to do so.

| | |
|---|---|
| tetralogy of Fallot | Laennec's cirrhosis |
| Cheyne-Stokes respiration | Osler's phenomenon |
| Dupuytren's contracture | Bell's palsy |
| Hirschsprung's disease | Tietze's syndrome |
| Sydenham's cough | Escherich's reflex |
| Shiga's bacillus | Biermer's anemia |
| MacCallum's patch | |

See also *Note* in introduction.


**DON'T**  capitalize most words **derived** from eponymic names.

Parkinson's disease **but** parkinsonism
Addison's disease **but** addisonian
Cushing's syndrome **but** cushingoid facies

**NOTE.**  *Syndrome names in the nonpossessive form are idiomatically preceded by* the.

Anton's syndrome **but** the Guillain-Barré syndrome

# 12 EPONYMS

## 12—3    INCISIONS, PROCEDURES, AND OPERATIONS

**_DO_**     capitalize an eponym that refers to a particular surgical incision or operative procedure and show the possessive ('s) when appropriate to do so.

Eloesser flap
Girdlestone-Taylor procedure
Billroth II gastric resection
Pfannenstiel incision
Buck's operation
Esser graft
Maisonneuve's amputation
Roux's anastomosis

## 12—4    MICROBIOLOGY

**_DO_**     capitalize an eponym that refers to a particular microorganism and show the possessive ('s) when appropriate to do so.

Epstein-Barr virus
Zimmermann virus
Whitmore's bacillus
Dutton's spirochete
Escherich's bacillus

## 12—5    PHARMACOLOGY

**_DO_**     capitalize an eponym that refers to a particular pharmaceutical, drug, or substance and show the possessive ('s).

Bamberger's fluid
Pover's powder
Fothergill's pills
Seignette's salt
Weichardt's antikenotoxin

## 12—6   PLURALS

See Chapter 25, *Plural Forms*, Rule 25–6.

## 12—7   POSITIONS

***DO***   capitalize an eponym that refers to a particular patient position for a surgical or diagnostic procedure and use the possessive ('s) when appropriate to do so.

| | |
|---|---|
| Trendelenburg's position | Caldwell position |
| Gaynor-Hart position | Fowler's position |
| Sims' position | Rose's position |

## 12—8   SIGNS, TESTS, AND OTHER THEORETICAL KNOWLEDGE

***DO***   capitalize an eponym that refers to a particular sign, test, law, theory, formula, constant, reaction, and so forth, and show the possessive ('s) when appropriate to do so.

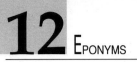

# 12 EPONYMS

Babinski's sign
Hoffmann's reflex
Widowitz's sign
Planck's constant
Pfeiffer's phenomenon
(or reaction)
Wassermann test
(or reaction)
Pignet's formula

Apgar score
Tyndall effect
Waters' view
Buergi's theory
Krebs' cycle
Maurer's dots
Bowie's stain
Dubois' method
Coombs' test

## 12—9    SURGICAL AND OTHER INSTRUMENTS

**_DO_**    capitalize an eponym but **do not show the possessive** ('s) when it describes surgical and diagnostic instruments, materials, solutions, and so forth.

Mayo scissors
Richard retractors
Foley catheter
Liston-Stille forceps
Starr-Edwards valve

Gigli saw
Glassman clamp
Castroviejo knife
DeBakey prosthesis
Crozat appliance

## 12—10    TREATMENT

**_DO_**    capitalize an eponym that describes a particular treatment or test and show the possessive ('s).

Balfour's treatment
Dubois' method
Fliess' therapy
Rollier's radiation
Ebstein's diet

# 13

# Exclamation

# Mark

## 13—1  DASHES

**_DO_**    use dashes to set off an exclamation within a sentence. The exclamation mark should be placed before the closing dash.

The new staff physician — I couldn't understand him! — dictated as though he was chewing peanuts.

**_DO_**    use an exclamation point at the end of an exclamatory sentence using a closing dash.

STAT transcription service delivers the reports—on time!

## 13—2  PARENTHESES

**DON'T**    use an exclamation point before the closing parenthesis unless it refers to the parenthetical item and the sentence ends with a different mark of punctuation. See example on next page.

Be sure to send the medical report to the state hospital in Washburn, Maine (not Washburn, Wisconsin!).

**_DO_**    use an exclamation point outside the closing parenthesis if the phrase in parentheses is to be incorporated at the end of a sentence.

What a terrific outcome (a once in a lifetime opportunity)!

## 13—3    PUNCTUATION

**_DO_**    use an exclamation point following a word, phrase, clause, or sentence to indicate a forceful statement or great surprise.

Physicians have had enough of governmental interference in medical practice!

No!

Congratulations! Your baby is completely healthy.

**_DO_**    use a comma or period if the exclamation is mild.

Yes, tell Ms. Seitz to come to the office tomorrow.

Well, I think you had better deliver this in person.

## 13—4    QUOTATION MARKS

**_DO_**    use an exclamation mark outside the closing quotation mark when it applies to the entire sentence.

She keeps telling me, "I'm leaving this job"!

**_DO_**    use quotation marks outside the closing exclamation mark when a quoted sentence stands alone or is at the beginning or end of a sentence.

"I won't accept that as payment in full!" I told him.

## 13—5    SPACING

**_DO_**    use two spaces after an exclamation mark at the end of a sentence.

*NOTE.    There is no space after an exclamation mark when another mark of punctuation (closing quotation mark, parenthesis, or dash) immediately follows.*

**129**

# 14

# HISTORY

# AND

# PHYSICAL

# FORMAT

## INTRODUCTION

**_DO_**     use the formats and standard outlines preferred in your locality and/or hospital facility. Remember that appearance and ease of readability are important considerations.

## 14—1   CONTINUATION SHEETS

**_DO_**     type headings for page 2 and subsequent pages using the format preferred by your employer and/or hospital facility. This would include the patient's name, medical record number, page number, and other optional statistical information (name of attending physician).

**_DO_**      type flush with the left margin or use a horizontal format.

Robert J. Newton
#45700
Page 2

*or*

Robert J. Newton    #45700        Page 2

**_DO_**      type *continued* on the bottom of each incomplete sheet beginning with the first page when there is more than one sheet.

## 14—2   DATES

**_DO_**      use the date the material was dictated, *not* the day it was transcribed in hospital transcription.

**_DO_**      spell out the date in full in either the traditional or the military style.

December 22, 199x (traditional)
22 December 199x (British and military)

**_DO_**      type the dates of dictation and transcription at the end of the history and physical and other report formats on two lines below the reference initials.

lwc:dt
D: 10-12-9x (D indicates the date dictated)
T: 10-13-9x (T indicates the date transcribed)

## 14—3    FORMAT STYLES

### Full Block Format (Fig. 14–1)

**_DO_**    begin all lines including headings and subheadings at the left margin.

**Figure 14–1.** Example of a history and physical typed in full block format.

de Mars, Verna Marie

Cortland M. Struthers, M. D.

HISTORY

CHIEF COMPLAINT:

Prolapse and bleeding after each bowel movement for the past 3–4 months.

PRESENT ILLNESS:

This 68-year-old white female says she usually has three bowel movements a day in small amounts, and there has been a recent change in the frequency, size, and type of bowel movement she has been having. She is also having some pain and irritation in this area. She has had no previous anorectal surgery or rectal infection. She denies any blood in the stool itself.

PAST HISTORY:

ILLNESSES:  The patient had polio at age 8, from which she made a remarkable recovery. Apparently, she was paralyzed in both lower extremities but now has adequate use of these. She has had no other serious illnesses.

ALLERGIES:  ALLERGIC TO PENICILLIN. She denies any other drug or food allergies.

MEDICATIONS:  None.

OPERATIONS:  Herniorrhaphy, 25 years ago.

SOCIAL:  She does not smoke or drink. She lives with her husband, who is an invalid and for whom she provides care. She is a retired municipal court judge.

(continued)

133

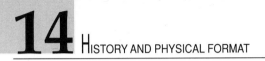

Verna Marie de Mars
#62789
Page 2

<u>FAMILY</u> <u>HISTORY</u>:

One brother died of cancer of the throat; another has cancer of the kidney.

<u>REVIEW</u> <u>OF</u> <u>SYSTEMS</u>:

SKIN: No rashes or jaundice.

HEENT: Unremarkable.

CR: No history of chest pain, shortness of breath, or pedal edema. She has had some mild hypertension in the past but is not under any medical supervision, nor is she taking any medication for this.

GI: Weight is stable. See <u>Present</u> <u>Illness</u>.

OB-GYN: Gravida II Para II. Climacteric at age 46, no sequelae.

EXTREMITIES: No edema.

NEUROLOGIC: Unremarkable.

PHYSICAL EXAMINATION

<u>GENERAL</u>:

This is a 68-year-old, well-developed, well-nourished, slightly obese white woman in no acute distress. She is alert and oriented to time, place, and person.

<u>VITAL</u> <u>SIGNS</u>:

Pulse: 76/min. Blood pressure: 130/80. Respirations: 12. Temperature: 99°.

<u>HEENT</u>:

EYES: Pupils equal and react to light and accommodation. EOMs intact. Sclerae white. Fundi not visualized.

EARS: Hearing and drums are normal.

MOUTH: The teeth are in poor repair. Several bridges are present. The tongue protrudes in the midline with some questionable deviation to the right. Uvula projects upward on elicitation of the gag reflex. No lesions of the mucous membranes.

(continued)

Verna Marie de Mars
#62789
Page 3

## NECK:

Supple with some limitation of motion to the right. No masses present. The carotid pulsations are equal with no bruit. There is no neck vein distention and no thyromegaly. The trachea is deviated slightly to the right.

## CHEST:

No increase in AP diameter.

LUNGS: Clear to P&A.

HEART: Quiet precordium. Normal sinus rhythm without murmurs, rubs, or gallops. Heart sounds appear normal and split physiologically. No S-4 heard.

## ABDOMEN:

Flat, without scars. No organomegaly. Liver, kidneys, and spleen not palpable. Tympanic to percussion. The bowel sounds are normoactive.

## PELVIC:

Deferred.

## RECTAL:

On anoscopy, there is an exophytic, soft, easily movable mass encompassing one-half the circumference of the rectum directly at the dentate line. Full sigmoidoscopic examination to 25 cm was unremarkable.

## EXTREMITIES:

Range of motion is within normal limits. No pedal edema. All pulses appear equal and full bilaterally. No evidence of chronic arterial or venous disease.

## NEUROLOGIC:

Cranial nerves II-XII appear grossly intact. There are no pathologic reflexes demonstrated. Reflexes within normal limits.

(continued)

Verna Marie de Mars
#62789
Page 4

IMPRESSION:

Rectal tumor.

---

Cortland M. Struthers, M.D.

jrt
D: 5-17-9x
T: 5-20-9x

---

Indented Format (Fig. 14–2)

**_DO_**      indent subtopics 3 to 5 spaces under the main topics.

**_DO_**      begin all data single spaced on the same line as the topic or subtopic.

**_DO_**      begin the first and second lines of each paragraph under a major heading 23 to 27 spaces from the left margin. Third and subsequent lines should be brought back to the left margin (as long as they clear the outline — if only a few words block under first two lines).

SOCIAL:    She does not smoke or drink. She lives with her husband, who is an invalid and for whom she provides care. She is a retired municipal court judge.

*or*

SOCIAL:    She does not smoke or drink. She lives with her husband, who is an invalid. She is a retired municipal court judge.

**Figure 14–2.** Example of a history and physical typed using indented format.

---

de Mars, Verna Marie

Cortland M. Struthers, M. D.

HISTORY

CHIEF COMPLAINT:      Prolapse and bleeding after each bowel movement for the past 3–4 months.

PRESENT ILLNESS:      This 68-year-old white female says she usually has three bowel movements a day in small amounts, and there has been a recent change in the frequency, size, and type of bowel movement she has been having. She is also having some pain and irritation in this area. She has had no previous anorectal surgery or rectal infection. She denies any blood in the stool itself.

PAST HISTORY:

    ILLNESSES:      The patient had polio at age 8, from which she made a remarkable recovery. Apparently, she was paralyzed in both lower extremities but now has adequate use of these. She has had no other serious illnesses.

    ALLERGIES:      ALLERGIC TO PENICILLIN. She denies any other drug or food allergies.

    MEDICATIONS:      None.

    OPERATIONS:      Herniorrhaphy, 25 years ago.

    SOCIAL:      She does not smoke or drink. She lives with her husband, who is an invalid and for whom she provides care. She is a retired municipal court judge.

FAMILY HISTORY:      One brother died of cancer of the throat; another has cancer of the kidney.

REVIEW OF SYSTEMS:

    SKIN:      No rashes or jaundice.

    HEENT:      Unremarkable.

(continued)

Verna Marie de Mars
#62789
Page 2

CR: No history of chest pain, shortness of breath, or pedal edema. She has had some mild hypertension in the past but is not under any medical supervision, nor is she taking any medication for this.

GI: Weight is stable. See Present Illness.

OB-GYN: Gravida II Para II. Climacteric at age 46, no sequelae.

EXTREMITIES: No edema.

NEUROLOGIC: Unremarkable.

_____
Cortland M. Struthers, M. D.

jrt
D: 5-17-9x
T: 5-20-9x


PHYSICAL EXAMINATION

GENERAL: This is a 68-year-old, well-developed, well-nourished, slightly obese white woman in no acute distress. She is alert and oriented to time, place, and person.

VITAL SIGNS: Pulse: 76/min. Blood pressure: 130/80. Respirations: 12. Temperature: 99°.

HEENT:

EYES: Pupils equal and react to light and accommodation. EOMs intact. Sclerae white. Fundi not visualized.

EARS: Hearing and drums are normal.

MOUTH: The teeth are in poor repair. Several bridges are present. The tongue protrudes in the midline with some questionable deviation to the right. Uvula projects upward on elicitation of the gag reflex. No lesions of the mucous membranes.

(continued)

Verna Marie de Mars
#62789
Page 3

NECK: Supple with some limitation of motion to the right. No masses present. The carotid pulsations are equal with no bruit. There is no neck vein distention and no thyromegaly. The trachea is deviated slightly to the right.

CHEST: No increase in AP diameter.

LUNGS: Clear to P&A.

HEART: Quiet precordium. Normal sinus rhythm without murmurs, rubs, or gallops. Heart sounds appear normal and split physiologically. No S-4 heard.

ABDOMEN: Flat, without scars. No organomegaly. Liver, kidneys, and spleen not palpable. Tympanic to percussion. The bowel sounds are normoactive.

PELVIC: Deferred.

RECTAL: On anoscopy, there is an exophytic, soft, easily movable mass encompassing one-half the circumference of the rectum directly at the dentate line. Full sigmoidoscopic examination to 25 cm was unremarkable.

EXTREMITIES: Range of motion is within normal limits. No pedal edema. All pulses appear equal and full bilaterally. No evidence of chronic arterial or venous disease.

NEUROLOGIC: Cranial nerves II-XII appear grossly intact. There are no pathologic reflexes demonstrated. Reflexes within normal limits.

IMPRESSION: Rectal tumor.

_____

Cortland M. Struthers, M. D.

jrt
D: 5-17-9x
T: 5-20-9x

Modified Block Format (Fig. 14–3)

**_DO_**       indent subtopics 3 to 5 spaces under the main topics.

**_DO_**       begin all data single-spaced on the same line as the topic or subtopic. Tabulate 23 spaces from the left margin.

CHIEF COMPLAINT:       Prolapse and bleeding
                       after each bowel movement
                       for the past 3–4 months.

PRESENT ILLNESS:       This 68-year-old white female says
                       she usually has three bowel
                       movements a day in small amounts,
                       and there has been a recent change in
                       frequency, size, and type of bowel
                       movement she has been having. She
                       is also having some pain and irritation
                       in this area. She has had no previous
                       anorectal surgery or rectal infection.
                       She denies any blood in the stool itself.

**Figure 14–3.** Example of a history and physical typed using modified block format.

---

de Mars, Verna Marie

Cortland M. Struthers, M. D.

                       HISTORY

<u>CHIEF</u> <u>COMPLAINT</u>:       Prolapse and bleeding after each bowel
                       movement for the past 3–4 months.

<u>PRESENT</u> <u>ILLNESS</u>:       This 68-year-old white female says she
                       usually has three bowel movements a
                       day in small amounts, and there has
                       been a recent change in the frequency,
                       size, and type of bowel movement she
                       has been having. She is also having
                       some pain and irritation in this area. She
                       has had no previous anorectal surgery or
                       rectal infection. She denies any blood in
                       the stool itself.

 (continued)

Verna Marie de Mars
#62789
Page 2

PAST HISTORY:

ILLNESSES: The patient had polio at age 8, from which she made a remarkable recovery. Apparently, she was paralyzed in both lower extremities but now has adequate use of these. She has had no other serious illnesses.

ALLERGIES: ALLERGIC TO PENICILLIN. She denies any other drug or food allergies.

MEDICATIONS: None.

OPERATIONS: Herniorrhaphy, 25 years ago.

SOCIAL: She does not smoke or drink. She lives with her husband, who is an invalid and for whom she provides care. She is a retired municipal court judge.

FAMILY HISTORY: One brother died of cancer of the throat; another has cancer of the kidney.

REVIEW OF SYSTEMS:

SKIN: No rashes or jaundice.

HEENT: Unremarkable.

CR: No history of chest pain, shortness of breath, or pedal edema. She has had some mild hypertension in the past but is not under any medical supervision nor is she taking any medication for this.

GI: Weight is stable. See Present Illness.

OB-GYN: Gravida II Para II. Climacteric at age 46, no sequelae.

EXTREMITIES: No edema.

(continued)

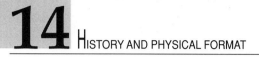

Verna Marie de Mars
#62789
Page 3

NEUROLOGIC: Unremarkable.

---

Cortland M. Struthers, M. D.

jrt
D: 5-17-9x
T: 5-20-9x

## PHYSICAL EXAMINATION

GENERAL:

This is a 68-year-old, well-developed, well-nourished, slightly obese white woman in no acute distress. She is alert and oriented to time, place, and person.

VITAL SIGNS:

Pulse: 76/min. Blood pressure: 130/80. Respirations: 12. Temperature: 99°.

HEENT:

EYES:

Pupils equal and react to light and accommodation. EOMs intact. Sclerae white. Fundi not visualized.

EARS:

Hearing and drums are normal.

MOUTH:

The teeth are in poor repair. Several bridges are present. The tongue protrudes in the midline with some questionable deviation to the right. Uvula projects upward on elicitation of the gag reflex. No lesions of the mucous membranes.

NECK:

Supple with some limitation of motion to the right. No masses present. The carotid pulsations are equal with no bruit. There is no neck vein distention and no thyromegaly. The trachea is deviated slightly to the right.

(continued)

Verna Marie de Mars
#62789
Page 4

| | |
|---|---|
| CHEST: | No increase in AP diameter. |
| LUNGS: | Clear to P&A. |
| HEART: | Quiet precordium. Normal sinus rhythm without murmurs, rubs, or gallops. Heart sounds appear normal and split physiologically. No S-4 heard. |
| ABDOMEN: | Flat, without scars. No organomegaly. Liver, kidneys, and spleen not palpable. Tympanic to percussion. The bowel sounds are normoactive. |
| PELVIC: | Deferred. |
| RECTAL: | On anoscopy, there is an exophytic, soft, easily movable mass encompassing one-half the circumference of the rectum directly at the dentate line. Full sigmoidoscopic examination to 25 cm was unremarkable. |
| EXTREMITIES: | Range of motion is within normal limits. No pedal edema. All pulses appear equal and full bilaterally. No evidence of chronic arterial or venous disease. |
| NEUROLOGICAL: | Cranial nerves II-XII appear grossly intact. There are no pathological reflexes demonstrated. Reflexes within normal limits. |
| IMPRESSION: | Rectal tumor. |

_____

Cortland M. Struthers, M. D.

jrt
D: 5-17-9x
T: 5-20-9x

Run-on Format (Fig. 14–4)

| | |
|---|---|
| **_DO_** | begin all data single-spaced on the same line as the topic or subtopic. Tabulations, underlining, and double spacing are lessened or eliminated entirely in run-on format. |

**Figure 14–4.**   History and physical typed in run-on format.

---

de Mars, Verna Marie

Cortland M. Struthers, M. D.

### HISTORY

CHIEF COMPLAINT: Prolapse and bleeding after each bowel movement for the past 3–4 months.

PRESENT ILLNESS: This 68-year-old white female says she usually has three bowel movements a day in small amounts, and there has been a recent change in the frequency, size, and type of bowel movement she has been having. She is also having some pain and irritation in this area. She has had no previous anorectal surgery or rectal infection. She denies any blood in the stool itself.

PAST HISTORY:

ILLNESSES: The patient had polio at age 8, from which she made a remarkable recovery. Apparently, she was paralyzed in both lower extremities but now has adequate use of these. She has had no other serious illnesses.

ALLERGIES: ALLERGIC TO PENICILLIN. She denies any other drug or food allergies.

MEDICATIONS: None.

OPERATIONS: Herniorrhaphy, 25 years ago.

SOCIAL: She does not smoke or drink. She lives with her husband, who is an invalid and for whom she provides care. She is a retired municipal court judge.

FAMILY HISTORY: One brother died of cancer of the throat, another has cancer of the kidney.

REVIEW OF SYSTEMS:

SKIN: No rashes or jaundice.

HEENT: Unremarkable.

CR: No history of chest pain, shortness of breath, or pedal edema. She has had some mild hypertension in the past but is not under any medical supervision, nor is she taking any medication for this.

(continued)

Verna Marie de Mars
#62789
Page 2

GI: Weight is stable. See <u>Present</u> <u>Illness</u>.
OB-GYN: Gravida II Para II. Climacteric at age 46, no sequelae.
EXTREMITIES: No edema.
NEUROLOGIC: Unremarkable.

PHYSICAL EXAMINATION

<u>GENERAL</u>: This is a 68-year-old, well-developed, well-nourished, slightly obese white woman in no acute distress. She is alert and oriented to time, place, and person.
<u>VITAL SIGNS</u>: Pulse: 76/min. Blood pressure: 130/80. Respirations: 12. Temperature: 99°.
<u>HEENT</u>:
EYES: Pupils equal and react to light and accommodation. EOMs intact. Sclerae white. Fundi not visualized.
EARS: Hearing and drums are normal.
MOUTH: The teeth are in poor repair. Several bridges are present. The tongue protrudes in the midline with some questionable deviation to the right. Uvula projects upward on elicitation of the gag reflex. No lesions of the mucous membranes.
<u>NECK</u>: Supple with some limitation of motion to the right. No masses present. The carotid pulsations are equal with no bruit. There is no neck vein distention and no thyromegaly. The trachea is deviated slightly to the right.
<u>CHEST</u>: No increase in AP diameter.
LUNGS: Clear to P&A.
HEART: Quiet precordium. Normal sinus rhythm without murmurs, rubs, or gallops. Heart sounds appear normal and split physiologically. No S-4 heard.
<u>ABDOMEN</u>: Flat, without scars. No organomegaly. Liver, kidneys, and spleen not palpable. Tympanic to percussion. The bowel sounds are normoactive.
PELVIC: Deferred.
<u>RECTAL</u>: On anoscopy, there is an exophytic, soft, easily movable mass encompassing one-half the circumference of the rectum directly at the dentate line. Full sigmoidoscopic examination to 25 cm was unremarkable.
<u>EXTREMITIES</u>: Range of motion is within normal limits. No pedal edema. All pulses appear equal and full bilaterally. No evidence of chronic arterial or venous disease.

(continued)

Verna Marie de Mars
#62789
Page 3

NEUROLOGIC:  Cranial nerves II-XII appear grossly intact. There are no pathologic reflexes demonstrated. Reflexes within normal limits.

IMPRESSION:  Rectal tumor.

_____

Cortland M. Struthers, M. D.

jrt
D: 5-17-9x
T:  5-20-9x

---

### Allergies

**_DO_**     type in all capitals and/or underline when the patient has allergies to food or drugs.

PAST HISTORY:    Illnesses:  The patient had polio at age 8, from which she has made a remarkable recovery. She was paralyzed in the right lower extremity and now has use of it. Allergies: <u>ALLERGIC</u> <u>TO</u> <u>PENICILLIN</u>. She denies any other drug or food allergies.

### Diagnosis

**_DO_**     spell out any terms dictated as abbreviations in the diagnosis portion of a history and physical.

DIAGNOSIS:  ASHD (incorrect)
DIAGNOSIS:  Arteriosclerotic heart disease (correct)

**_DO_** use numbering if dictated; it is optional if not dictated.

DIAGNOSES: Gastritis.
Pancreatitis.

*or*

DIAGNOSES:
1. Gastritis.
2. Pancreatitis.

## 14—4 HEADINGS

**_DO_** type all capitals for major headings followed by a colon. It is optional to underline or put the main topic on a line by itself.

PHYSICAL EXAMINATION:
There is marked hypertrophy of the nasal turbinates with obstruction of the airways. The conjunctivae were not injected. The tonsils were hypertrophic but did not appear actively infected. Lungs were clear.

## 14—5 INTERVAL HISTORY OR NOTE

A complete history and physical does not have to be completed on the patient for an interval history or note (Fig. 14–5), since this report is usually generated within a month after the patient's discharge from the hospital. The present complaint and interval history are emphasized in the report. The physical examination would include any new findings since the last examination and may also include a brief check on vital body systems. A more extensive examination would be done if the patient were readmitted to the hospital.

**Figure 14–5.** Example of an interval history typed in modified block style.

| | |
|---|---|
| Benita L. Martinez | March 17, 199x |
| 09-74-12 | William B. Dixon, M. D. |

## INTERVAL HISTORY

PRESENT COMPLAINT: This is a 45-year-old female who the first of March had a Roux-en-Y gastrojejunostomy done for a reflux bile gastritis. Postoperatively, she did moderately well; however, she began to evidence signs of anastomotic obstruction which got persistently worse. Upper GI series was done 4 days ago which showed an almost complete obstruction of the anastomosis. Patient is now being admitted for decompression of her stomach and revision of the gastrojejunostomy.

PAST HISTORY: Regional family; see old chart.

PHYSICAL EXAMINATION: Well-developed, well-nourished, but nervous, white female in no acute distress.

HEENT: Eyes: React to L&A. Ears: Canals and membranes normal. Nose: Negative. Neck: Supple with no masses, no enlargement of glands. Thyroid: Not palpable.

LUNGS: Clear to percussion and auscultation.

HEART: Rhythm and rate normal. No murmurs. No enlargements.

(continued)

Benita L. Martinez
#57621
Page 2

| | |
|---|---|
| ABDOMEN: | Recent bilateral subcostal incision, well healed. No other abdominal masses. |
| PELVIC: | Not done. |
| EXTREMITIES: | Negative. |
| IMPRESSION: | Gastrojejunal anastomotic obstructions. |
| ADVICE: | 1. Decompression by Levin tube. |
| | 2. Re-resection and anastomose tomorrow. |

William B. Dixon, M. D.

mlo
D: 3-17-9x
T: 3-20-9x

## 14—6   MARGINS

**_DO_**      use one-half inch to three-quarter inch right and left and bottom margins.

## 14—7 NUMBERING

***DO*** number all or none of the entries when typing if the dictator numbers some but not all items in a series. Be consistent.

MEDICATIONS: 1) Mylanta, 1 tsp ac.
2) Mellaril, 25 mg q.i.d. in liquid form.

## 14—8 OUTLINE

**DON'T** use abbreviations unless they are approved by your employer.

***DO***  type in main headings whether dictated or not and insert those subheadings as dictated. The following are standard headings:

History
Chief Complaint (abbreviated CC)
History of Present Illness (or History of
   Chief Complaint) abbreviated PI or HPI
Family History
Social History
Allergies
Habits
Past Medical History (abbreviated PH)
Review of Systems (abbreviated ROS)
General
Head, Eyes, Ears, Nose, Throat, Mouth,
   Teeth (or HEENT)
Cardiovascular
Respiratory or Cardiorespiratory (abbreviated CR)
Gastrointestinal (abbreviated GI)
Genitourinary (abbreviated GU)
Gynecologic (abbreviated GYN)
Neuropsychiatric (abbreviated NP)
Musculoskeletal (abbreviated MS)
Physical Examination (abbreviated PX or PE)
General Appearance
Vital Signs (abbreviated VS)
Skin
Head, Face, Neck. Head, Eyes, Ears, Nose, and
   Throat are abbreviated HEENT.
Eyes
Ears
Nose, Mouth, Throat, Teeth
Thorax, Breasts, Axillae
Heart
Lungs
Abdomen, Groin, Rectum, Anus, Genitalia
Back and Extremities
Neurologic
Mental Status (Psychiatric)
Diagnosis (Impression, Assessment, or Conclusion)
   abbreviated Dx or DX
Treatment (Recommendation) abbreviated TX or Tx
Plan

## 14—9    PAST AND PRESENT TENSE

**_DO_**    use the past tense in the past history portion of a report, in the discharge summary, or to discuss an expired patient.

**_DO_**    use present tense when describing the current illness or disease in the history and physical.

## 14—10    REFERENCE INITIALS

**_DO_**    use a double space below the typed signature line and type flush with the left margin.

**_DO_**    type the dictator's, signer's, and the typist's initials when the dictator differs from the person who signs the history and physical.

mjp/lrc/wpd            *or*            mjp:lrc:wpd

(Here, *mjp* stands for the dictator, *lrc* stands for the signer, and *wpd* stands for the typist.)

**DON'T**    use humorous or confusing combinations of reference initials.

crc (rather than cc)
db (rather than dmb)
dg (rather than dog)

## 14—11    SHORT-STAY RECORD

When a patient is admitted for 48 hours or less (diagnostic procedure or minor operative procedure), a shortened form of the history and physical examination record is acceptable in most hospitals (Fig. 14–6).

**Figure 14–6.** Example of a short-stay record typed in modified block format.

---

Roland, Jamie T.
543098

June 8, 199x

Copy:  Robert R. Shoemaker, M. D.

### SHORT-STAY RECORD

| | |
|---|---|
| HISTORY: | Patient is a 6-year-old male complaining of frequent episodes of tonsillitis. He missed several weeks of school this spring because of infections. He is a constant mouth breather. He snores loudly at night. He has constant nasal obstruction. There is no history of earaches. |
| PAST HISTORY: | There are no allergies. Bleeding history: None. Operations: None. Illnesses: None. Medications: Vitamins, iron. He has been on penicillin for resolution of symptoms. Family History: Noncontributory. |
| PHYSICAL EXAMINATION: | Skin: No rashes. EENT: Ears: TMs and canals appeared normal. Nose: Congested posteriorly but not anteriorly. Throat: Very large cryptic tonsils meeting in the midline. Neck: Numerous palpable nodes. |
| CHEST: | Lungs: Clear to percussion and auscultation. Heart: Not enlarged, normal sinus rhythm, no murmurs. |

(continued)

Jamie T. Roland
#543098
Page 2

| | |
|---|---|
| ABDOMEN: | Soft, nontender. |
| EXTREMITIES: | Full range of motion. |
| NEUROLOGIC: | Completely normal. |
| IMPRESSION: | Chronic hypertrophic tonsils and adenoids with recurrent infections. |
| RECOMMENDATION: | Tonsillectomy and adenoidectomy. |

_____

Peter Anthony Nelson, M. D.

sd
D: 6-8-9x
T: 6-8-9x

---

## 14—12    SIGNATURE LINE

**_DO_**    space 4 to 6 lines between the end of the report and the signature line.

**_DO_**    type the dictator's name. It is optional to insert a line for the signature.

## 14—13    SPACING OF HEADINGS

**_DO_**    use double spacing or a space and a half between the last line of one heading and the next heading. It is optional to use no space below the main topic. Headings not dictated should be inserted.

## 14—14   STATISTICAL DATA

***DO***   include the information and use the format preferred by your employer and/or hospital facility. The following is statistical data that may or may not be listed.

Patient's name
Age
Date of admission
Date of dictation
Medical record number
Hospital room number
Name of attending physician
Name of referring physician
Name(s) of anyone who is to receive a copy of
   the report

## 14—15   SUBHEADINGS

***DO***   type subheadings in all capitals or upper and lower case followed by a colon. It is optional to begin each subtopic on a separate line. Subheadings not dictated may be inserted but this too is optional.

HEENT:
EYES: Pupils are equal and react to light and accommodation.
EARS: Tympanic membranes are intact.
NOSE AND THROAT: Essentially unremarkable.

*or*

HEENT: Eyes: Pupils are equal and react to light and accommodation. Ears: Tympanic membranes are intact. Nose and throat: Essentially unremarkable.

## 14—16    TITLES

**_DO_**    center on the page and type in all capital letters. It is
optional to underline the title.

HISTORY
PHYSICAL EXAMINATION
HISTORY AND PHYSICAL

# 15

# HYPHEN

# USE AND

# WORD

# DIVISION

## INTRODUCTION

Hyphens are used primarily to aid the reader and avoid ambiguity. If your typing equipment automatically justifies margins, then hyphenation is out of your hands. But if the decision to divide words is yours, then the following rules are used as guides to clarity.

Please refer to Chapter 7, *Compounds,* for the many rules concerning the use of the hyphen in compound words.

# 15 HYPHEN USE AND WORD DIVISION

## 15—1    AMINO ACID SEQUENCES

***DO***    use a hyphen to separate the abbreviations for known amino acid sequences.

Lys-Asp-Gly

*NOTE. Unknown sequences are enclosed in parentheses and separated by commas.*

## 15—2    CHEMICAL ELEMENTS

***DO***    use a hyphen with letters or words describing chemical elements unless subscripts or superscripts are used instead.

Uranium-235    $U^{235}$

I-131         $I^{131}$    $^{131}I$    $^{18}F$

## 15—3    CHEMICAL FORMULAS

**_DO_**    use hyphens with prefixed locants (the chemical location in the molecule), chemical formulas, and conventions.

9-nitroanthra(1,9,4,10)bis(1)oxathiazone-2,7-bisdioxide

Leu-Glu-Pro-Ser-Thr-Ala

beta-sitosterol

cis-dichloroethene

2-hexanone

## 15—4    CLARITY

**_DO_**    use a hyphen to join two or more words used to describe a noun when clarity is required.

brown-bag lunch
small-town physician
long-awaited diagnosis

There was a soft-tissue lesion on the surface.
(The lesion is composed of soft tissue.)

**_DO_**   use a hyphen to join two or more words that have the force of a single modifier before a noun.

figure-of-eight sutures
self-addressed envelope
low-grade fever
self-inflicted knife wound
two-pack-a-day smoker
happy-go-lucky personality
well-known speaker
mouth-to-mouth resuscitation
through-and-through sutures
ill-defined tumor mass
up-to-date report
large-for-date fetus
non-English-speaking patient
diagnosis-related groups

She is a well-developed, well-nourished, 35-year-old black female.

She was seen today in final follow-up examination.

An end-to-end anastomosis was performed.

The resident consulted the alcoholism counselors on his two MAST-positive patients.

This is a very up-to-date reference for drug names.

**DON'T**   change the meaning of the dictator by attempting to clarify an expression.

"The gangrene was in the lower third of his leg."
NOT
"the lower one-third of his leg." This is too specific for the statement made.

**DON'T** use a hyphen when the compound follows the noun.

I want these records brought **up to date**.

She appears to be **well nourished**.

**DON'T** make a compound modifier with an adverb ending in *ly*.

That was a poorly dictated report.

She is a moderately obese waitress.

*DO* use a hyphen after a prefix when the unhyphenated word would have a different meaning.

re-infuse (infuse again)
re-treat (treat again)
re-creation (create again)

## 15—5    NUMBERS

*DO* hyphenate numbers 21 through 99 when they are written out.

Fifty-five medical transcriptionists attended the meeting last night.

Ninety-nine percent of the time I am confident of the diagnosis.

*DO* hyphenate spelled out fractions.

She has spent one-third of her life concerned about the appearance of this scar.

## 15—6    RANGE INDICATOR

**_DO_**

use the hyphen to take the place of the word _to_ or _through_, to identify numeric and alphabetic ranges.

take 100 mg Tylenol, 1–2 h.s.

the L2–5 vertebrae were involved

30–35 mEq

Rounds were made in Wards l–4.

practicing there from 1980–1989

checked the records from Blalock–Brownell

Check V2–V6 again.

We eliminated every diagnosis from A–Z.

Note the P-R interval.

**DON'T**

use a hyphen when one or both of the ranges contain a minus sign.

at a –2 to a –3 station

## 15—7   SUSPENDING HYPHEN

**DO**   use a suspending hyphen to connect a series of compound modifiers.

There were small- and large-sized cysts scattered throughout the parenchyma.

He has a two- or three-month convalescence ahead of him.

She had first- and second-degree burns on her upper extremities.

## 15—8   WORD DIVISION

**DO**   Use a hyphen to divide words at the end of a line. Avoid dividing words at the end of the line whenever you can. It takes time and breaks your rhythm and often confuses the reader. It is also easier to read and understand unhyphenated words. However, when you must divide a word, follow the rules provided here.

It is preferable to divide at certain points in order to obtain a more intelligible grouping of syllables. When in doubt about proper word division, check your dictionary or word-division manual. A word divided in error is just as incorrect as a word misspelled.

# 15 HYPHEN USE AND WORD DIVISION

## Rules for Dividing Words at the End of a Line

**_DO_**    divide English words **only** between syllables and in keeping with proper American pronunciation.

| | |
|---|---|
| knowl/edge | (*not* know/ledge) |
| liga/ture | (*not* lig/ature) |
| sepa/rate | (*not* sep/arate) |

dex/ter/ous    nom/i/na/tion    cel/lo/phane

**_DO_**    divide medical words either before a suffix, after a prefix, or between compounds.

dys/menorrhea    acro/phobia    ile/ostomy

**_DO_**    divide after a one-vowel syllable in the middle of a word.

organi/zation    regu/late    busi/ness

**_DO_**    divide between two vowels that appear together within the word.

cre/ative    retro/active    valu/able

**_DO_**    divide a word between doubled consonants, **but** divide a word root that **ends** with a double consonant between the root and the suffix.

| | | |
|---|---|---|
| swim/ming | occur/ring | control/ling |
| admit/ting | sug/gested | misspell/ing |
| fulfill/ment | | |

**_DO_**    divide a solid compound word between the elements of the compound.

over/riding      fiber/scope      off/spring
lack/luster       child/birth      gall/bladder

**_DO_**    divide a hyphenated compound word after the hyphen.

cross-/reference      extra-/oral

**_DO_**    divide a word with a prefix between the prefix and the root.

ante/natal      non/reactive      dys/phagia

**_DO_**    divide names between the given name and the surname. Include a middle initial with the given name; divide names preceded by long titles between the title and the name.

Annie P./Younger
Claude/Richey
Rear Admiral/John Wentworth
Mary Margaret/Smith

**_DO_**    avoid dividing dates. The only acceptable division of a date is between the comma (after the day) and the year.

September 1,/199X (correct)

September/ 1, 199X (incorrect)

Sep/tember 1, 199X (incorrect)

Rules for Avoiding Hyphenation

**DON'T** divide words of only one syllable or with fewer than six letters.

| | | | |
|---|---|---|---|
| pain | tumor | edema | weight |
| thought | unite | | |

> **NOTE.** *Even when* -ed *is added to some words, they still remain one syllable and cannot be divided.*

| | | |
|---|---|---|
| passed | trimmed | weighed |

**DON'T** divide words that will leave a confusing syllable on either line.

encom/pass (incorrect)
hot/test (incorrect)
wo/men (incorrect)

**DON'T** leave a one-letter syllable at the beginning or the end of a divided word. Do not divide a word unless you can leave a syllable of at least three characters (the last of which is the hyphen) on the upper line and you can carry a syllable of at least three characters (the last may be a punctuation mark) to the next line.

a-mount (incorrect)
bacteri-a (incorrect)
i-deal (incorrect)
pian-o (incorrect)

| | | |
|---|---|---|
| ad/ducent | de/capsulation | bi/lateral |

**DON'T**     divide names, other proper nouns, abbreviations, numbers, or contractions.

       William/son (incorrect)

       Ph.D.    ASCVHD    f.o.b.    can't    CMA-A    wouldn't

**_DO_**     write out a contraction to divide it.

       *NOTE.*    *Avoid writing contractions, in any case.*

       can/not       would/not

**DON'T**     divide identifying information from accompanying numbers.

| | | |
|---|---|---|
| 2 cm | page 84 | 6 lb 4 oz |
| December 1988 | | 1400 hours |

       Diagnoses: l. / Respiratory tract infection (incorrect)
       Diagnoses: / l. Respiratory tract infection (correct)

**DON'T**     divide a street address between the number and the street name but you may divide after the name of the street and before the word *street, avenue, circle,* and so forth.

       3821 /Ocean Street (incorrect)
       3821 Ocean/Street (correct)

       821 East Hazard/Road (correct)
       821 East/Hazard Road (incorrect)

**DON'T**   divide a word that would change its meaning when hyphenated.

        pre-position (to position again)
        re-form (to form again)
        re-mark (to mark again)
        re-treat (to treat again)
        re-creation (to create again)
        re-infuse (to infuse again)

**DON'T**   allow more than two consecutive lines to end in hyphens.

**DON'T**   divide at the end of the first line or at the end of the last full line in a paragraph.

**DON'T**   divide the last word on a page.

# 16

# LABORATORY

# TERMINOLOGY

# AND

# NORMAL

# VALUES

---

## 16—1    ABBREVIATIONS

See also Chapter 1, *Abbreviations and Symbols*.

**_DO_**    type a laboratory abbreviation if it is dictated.

RBC    WBC    BUN

**DON'T**    type an abbreviation if the dictator has used the full word without a number in the expression or sentence.

There was a high sodium level noted. (not "a high Na level")

**_DO_** use an abbreviation to refer to a test in a report or paper *after* it has been used once in its completely spelled-out form.

All newborns are routinely tested for phenylketonuria (PKU). As a result, the incidence of PKU as a cause of infant . . .

**DON'T** punctuate those scientific abbreviations written in a combination of upper- and lower-case letters.

IgG   mEq   pH   mOsm   Hb   Hct

## 16—2   BRIEF FORMS

**_DO_** add an "s" to a brief or short form for a laboratory term.

bands, stabs, segs, monos, lymphs, polys, eos, basos

## 16—3   CAPITALIZATION

**_DO_** use lower-case letters for metric symbols or abbreviations.

| kilogram | Kg (incorrect) | kg (correct) |
|---|---|---|
| milligram | Mg (incorrect) | mg (correct) |
| cubic millimeter | Cu mm (incorrect) | $mm^3$ (correct) |

*EXCEPTIONS. L for liter, C for Celsius, milliequivalent   meq (incorrect)   mEq (correct)*

## 16—4   COMPOUNDS

**DO**   use a hyphen to join a number to a word to form a coined compound phrase.

SMA-1      alpha-1      profile-1

**DO**   use a hyphen when a term is used as an adjective.

gram-positive organism      gram-negative stain

**DO**   use a hyphen to join a single letter to a word to form a coined compound.

T-cell leukemia

## 16—5   DECIMAL FRACTIONS

**DO**   type a whole number followed by a decimal point and one or two digits.

The arterial gases showed a pH of 7.45.

Urinalysis straw-colored, cloudy, pH 4.5, glucose 1+, acetone negative.

**DON'T**   type a whole number with a decimal point and zero, as it may be misread as a larger quantity.

Potassium 3.0 mEq/L (incorrect)
Potassium 3 mEq/L (correct)

**EXCEPTION.** *See Chapter 22, Rule 22–6.*

**_DO_** type specific gravity with four digits and a decimal point. Place the decimal point between the first and second digits even though the value may be dictated as "one zero," "one oh," or "ten." The normal range for specific gravity in urine is 1.015–1.025.

*Dictated*: Specific gravity "ten twenty."
*Transcribed*: Specific gravity 1.020.

*Dictated*: Specific gravity "one point zero three zero."
*Transcribed*: Specific gravity 1.030.

**_DO_** place a zero before a decimal point so it is not misread as a whole number.

.01 (incorrect)          0.01 (correct)

*Dictated*: point seventy-five percent basos
*Transcribed*: 0.75% basos

**_DO_** use a decimal fraction instead of a common fraction.

*Dictated*: Urinalysis revealed one quarter percent urine sugar.
*Transcribed*: Urinalysis revealed 0.25% urine sugar.

*Dictated*: Monocytes one and one-half per cent.
*Transcribed*: Monocytes 1.5%.

**DO**   use a period to separate a whole number from a decimal fraction.

> PTT 23.9. Globulins 2.8. Hematocrit 38.6 and hemoglobin 12.9.

## 16—6   EPONYMS

See also Chapter 12, *Eponyms*.

**DO**   capitalize an eponym that refers to a particular test and show the possessive ('s) when appropriate to do so.

> Wassermann's test (or reaction)
> Pfeiffer's phenomenon (or reaction)
> Salmonella-Shigella (agar)
> Eagle's basal (medium)
> Eijkman's lactose (broth)
> Pasteur's culture

## 16—7   GENUS

**DO**   abbreviate the genus (but not the species) after the genus has been used once in the text.

> The report was negative for Escherichia coli. We had expected to find E. coli . . .

**DO**   abbreviate the genus (but not the species) with a period.

> E. coli (Escherichia coli)
> H. influenzae (Haemophilus influenzae)

**DON'T**    abbreviate the genus when used alone without the species name.

His mycoplasma serology will not be repeated.

## 16—8    HYPHEN

*DO*    join a number to a word to form a coined compound phrase.

SMA-1        alpha-1        profile-1

*EXCEPTION.*    T3 or $T_3$    T4 or $T_4$

*DO*    use the hyphen to take the place of the word *to* identify numeric and alphabetic ranges.

30–35 mEq

**DON'T**    divide identifying information from accompanying numbers

Hgb 14.8.    pH 7.42.    CPK 716.

## 16—9    LOWER-CASE AND UPPER-CASE LETTERS

**DON'T**    use periods with scientific abbreviations that include upper-case and lower-case letters.

The arterial gases showed a pH of 7.45.

## 16—10    METRIC SYSTEM

See Chapter 21, *Metric System.*

## 16—11    NUMBERS

***DO***    use Arabic numerals to express laboratory values.

PTT 23.9. Globulins 2.8. Hematocrit 38.6 and hemoglobin 12.9.

WBC 3.8 thousand or WBC 3,800 or WBC 3800

***DO***    use commas to group numbers in units of three.

platelets 250,000; wbc 15,000

**DON'T**    use commas with the metric system or with decimals.

1000 ml (correct)
1 000 ml (a space is correct)
1,000 ml (incorrect)

***DO***    use figures when numbers are used directly with symbols or abbreviations.

pH 6.5    pO2    $pO_2$    pCO2    $pCO_2$

***DO***    leave a space between the number and the abbreviation.

IgA  60

**EXCEPTION.** *The Western Blot HIV AIDS test shows no space between the number and alpha character.*

Bands present at p24 and p55.
Bands present at p24, gp160.

**DO**      use figures with metric abbreviations

7 ml     20 kg     1 L

**DO**      use figures and symbols when writing plus or minus with a number.

1+ protein

## 16—12    PLURAL FORMS WITH LABORATORY ABBREVIATIONS

See also Rule 16–2, Brief Forms.

**DO**      use an apostrophe to form the plurals of lower case abbreviations and abbreviations that include periods.

There were elevated wbc's.

**DON'T**    use an apostrophe with other plural abbreviations.

The patient's white blood count was 4.8 thousand with 58% segs,
7% bands, 24% lymphs, 8% monos, 1% eos, and 2% basos.

## 16—13    PUNCTUATION WITH LABORATORY ABBREVIATIONS

***DO***    write most abbreviations in full capital letters without punctuation.

PKU   BUN   CBC   WBC   RBC

**DON'T**    punctuate those scientific abbreviations written in a combination of upper- and lower-case letters.

pH   Hb   Hgb   mEq   mOsm

***DO***    use commas when multiple related laboratory test results are reported.

Phosphorus 5.2, BUN 30, creatinine 1.4.
WBC 12.4 with 69 segs, 5 stabs.

*NOTE.* *It is optional to use commas to separate a laboratory value from the test it describes.*

Creatinine 1.4. Creatinine, 1.4. *or* Creatinine: 1.4.

*NOTE.* *For the sake of clarity in some instances it is wise to insert a colon. For example, $CO_2$: 24; $pCO_2$: 35. The numbers tend to run together when a colon is omitted.*

***DO***    use periods to separate unrelated laboratory test results.

White blood count 8,100. Potassium 3.3. SGOT 20. Albumin 4.4.

**DON'T**   separate sets of words incorrectly.

Serum electrolytes alkaline, phosphatase BUN, creatinine, glucose and calcium will be checked. (incorrect)

Serum electrolytes, alkaline phosphatase, BUN, creatinine, glucose, and calcium will be checked. (correct)

## 16—14   RATIOS

**DO**   use a colon to express ratios in which the colon takes the place of the word *to*.

The solution was diluted 1:100.
We had a 2:1 mix.

## 16—15   ROMAN NUMERALS

**DON'T**   use a type font that is sans serif (e.g., Chicago) because the capital letter I needed for Roman numerals looks like the number one.

**DO**   use Roman numerals with typical non-counting or non-mathematical listings.

Factor      missing Factor VII (blood factor)

Papanicolaou smears can be reported as Class I through Class V or by Cervical Intraepithelial Neoplasia (CIN) Classes I through III.

## 16—16   SHORT FORMS

See also Rule 16–2, *Brief Forms*

**_DO_**     type the short form, or brief form, when dictated if it does not violate any of the rules listed in 16–1.

> Pap smear (Papanicolaou)
> sed rate (sedimentation rate)
> lymphs (lymphocytes)
> monos (monocytes)
> eos (eosinophiles)
> basos (basophiles)
> alk. phos. (alkaline phosphatase)
> chem profile (chemistry profile)

## 16—17   SLASH

**_DO_**     use a slash in writing certain technical terms. The slash sometimes substitutes for the word *per* in laboratory terms.

> *Dictated*: The lumbar puncture showed one white blood cell per cubic millimeter.
> *Transcribed*: The lumbar puncture showed one white blood cell per cubic millimeter.
> *Alternative form*: 1 wbc/cu mm.

**DON'T**   use a slash to express a ratio.

> 1/20,000 (incorrect)
> 1:20,000 (correct)

## 16—18    SPECIFIC GRAVITY

**_DO_**       type specific gravity with four digits and a decimal point placed between the first and second digits even though the value may be dictated as "one zero," "one oh," or "ten."

*Dictated*: Specific gravity "ten twenty."
*Transcribed*: Specific gravity 1.020.

*Dictated*: Specific gravity "one point zero three zero."
*Transcribed*: Specific gravity 1.030.

## 16—19    STAINS

**_DO_**       type the word Gram with a capital G when indicating Gram's stain, method, or solution, since it is the last name of Hans Christian Joachim Gram. However, when Gram is used as a compound word, it begins with a lower-case g.

Gram's stain
gram-negative (means the specimen loses the stain)
gram-positive (means the specimen retains the stain)

## 16—20    SUBSCRIPT AND SUPERSCRIPT

**_DO_**       use numeric subscripts and capital letters when typing human blood groups or referring to thyroid tests.

Mrs. James's blood group test showed she is $A_2B$ positive.

The patient's $T_4$ was in the mid range of 7.1.

**NOTE.** *Except for mathmatical exponents ($10^5$), these expressions can be typed on the same line if your typing equipment is not capable of printing small numbers above or below the line.*

## 16—21    SYMBOLS

*DO*     use symbols only when they occur in immediate association with a number or another abbreviation.

| | |
|---|---|
| 4–5 | four to five |
| 2+ | two plus |
| diluted 1:10 | diluted one to ten |
| –2 | minus two |
| nocturia x 2 | nocturia times two |
| 25 mg/hr | twenty-five milligrams per hour |
| 35 mg% | thirty-five milligrams percent |

*DO*     leave a space between the number and the abbreviation.

50ml (incorrect)          50 ml (correct)

**DON'T**  leave a space between the number or abbreviation and a symbol.

| | |
|---|---|
| 50 % (incorrect) | 50% (correct) |
| 46 mg % (incorrect) | 46 mg% (correct) |

**_DO_**  be consistent when typing the percent sign even if the dictator dictates the first percent but does not dictate the rest of the percent symbols in a series of related tests.

The triglycerides were high at 646 mg% and cholesterol 283 mg%.

Blood sugar was 46 mg%.

The patient had a white blood count of 4.8 thousand with 58% segs, 7% bands, 24% lymphs, 8% monos, 1% eos, and 2% basos.

**_DO_**  use figures and symbols when writing plus or minus with a number.

1+ protein

**DON'T**  pluralize symbols.

| | | |
|---|---|---|
| kilograms | kgs (incorrect) | kg (correct) |
| meters | ms (incorrect) | m (correct) |

## 16—22    VALUES

Normal values vary from one laboratory to another, depending on types of equipment, so the figures listed in Table 16–1 are approximate.

## Table 16–1.  Normal Values for Laboratory Tests

**Blood Chemistries**

| | |
|---|---|
| A/G ratio (albumin/globulin ratio) | 1.1 to 2.3 |
| albumin | 3.0 to 5.0 grams/dl |
| BUN (blood urea nitrogen) | 10.0 to 26.0 mg/dl |
| Ca (calcium) | 8.5 to 10.5 mg/dl |
| cholesterol | 150 to 250 mg/dl |
| creatinine | 0.7 to 1.5 mg/dl |
| electrolytes | |
|   bicarb, serum (bicarbonate) | 23 to 29 mEq/liter |
|   cl (chlorides) | 96 to 106 mEq/liter |
|   GGTP (gamma-glutamyl transpeptidase) | 8.0 to 35.0 milliunits/ml |
|   K (potassium) | 3.5 to 5.0 mEq/liter |
|   magnesium, serum | 1.5 to 2.5 mEq/liter |
|   Na (sodium) | 136 to 145 mEq/liter |
|   phosphate | 3.0 to 4.5 mg/dl |
| globulin | 1.5 to 3.7 grams/dl |
| glucose | 60 to 100 mg/dl |
| immunoglobulins, serum | |
|   IgA | 60 to 333 mg/dl |
|   IgD | 0.5 to 3.0 mg/dl |
|   IgE | greater than 500 ng/ml |
|   IgG | 550 to 1900 mg/dl |
|   IgM | 45 to 145 mg/dl |
| iron, serum | 75 to 175 µg/dl |
| lipids | |
|   phospholipids | 60 to 350 mg/dl |
|   serum, total | 450 to 1000 mg/dl |
| lipoprotein cholesterol | |
|   high-density (HDL) | 26 to 63 mg/dl |
|   very low-density (VLDL) | 6 to 40 mg/dl |
|   low-density (LDL) | 105 to 213 mg/dl |
| liver functions | |
|   ACP (acid phosphatase) | |
|   ALP (alkaline phosphatase, serum) | 20 to 90 milliunits/ml |
|   bilirubin | 0.3 to 1.1 mg/dl |
|   LDH (lactate dehydrogenase) | 80 to 120 units/ml |
|   AST (aspartate amino transferase) SGOT (serum glutamic-oxaloacetic transaminase) | 0 to 19 milliunits/ml |
|   ALT (alamine amino transferase) SGPT (serum glutamic-pyruvic transaminase) | 0 to 17 milliunits/ml |
| total protein | 6.0 to 8.0 grams/dl |
| triglycerides, serum | 40 to 150 mg/dl |
| uric acid | 2.2 to 7.7 mg/dl |

*Table continued on following page*

### Table 16–1. Normal Values for Laboratory Tests *Continued*

**Blood Gases**

| | |
|---|---|
| $O_2$ (oxygen) | 15 to 24 vol. % |
| $CO_2$ (carbon dioxide) | 22 to 30 mmol/liter |
| $PO_2$ or $pO_2$ (oxygen partial pressure) | 75 to 100 mm Hg |
| $PCO_2$ or $pCO_2$ (carbon dioxide partial pressure) | 32 to 35 mm Hg |

**Hematology**

| | |
|---|---|
| CBC (complete blood count) | |
| WBC (white blood count or cells) | 4,200 to 10,000 |
| RBC (red blood count or cells) | Males 4.6 to 6.2 million/cu mm |
| | Females 4.2 to 5.4 million/cu mm |
| HGB or Hgb (hemoglobin) | Males 14 to 18 grams/dl |
| | Females 12 to 16 grams/dl |
| HCT or Hct (hematocrit) | Males 40 to 54 ml/dl |
| | Females 37 to 47 ml/dl |
| Indices | |
| MCV (mean corpuscular volume) | 80 to 105 microns |
| MCH (mean corpuscular hemoglobin) | 27 to 31 UUG |
| MCHC (mean corpuscular hemoglobin concentration) | 32 to 36% |
| Differential | |
| polys (polymorphonuclear neutrophils) referred to as: segs, stabs, bands | 54 to 62% |
| lymphs (lymphocytes) | 25 to 33% |
| eos or eosin (eosinophils) | 1 to 3% |
| monos (monocytes) | 3 to 7% |
| basos (basophils) | 0 to 0.75% |

*Note*: "Shift to the left" means there are increased numbers of immature neutrophils (band forms, not lobulations). Sometimes this indicates an infection.

Morphology
aniso (anisocytosis)
poik (poikilocytosis)
macro (macrocytic)
micro (microcytic)
hypochromia

**Table 16–1. Normal Values for Laboratory Tests** *Continued*

Morphology *continued*

| | |
|---|---|
| platelets | 150,000 to 350,000/cu mm |
| reticulocytes | 25,000 to 75,000/cu mm |

Coagulation Group

| | |
|---|---|
| ESR or Sed Rate (sedimentation rate) | Males 0 to 5 mm in 1 hr |
|    Wintrobe method: | Females 0 to 15 mm in 1 hr |
|    Westergren method: | Males 0 to 15 mm in 1 hr |
| | Females 0 to 20 mm in 1 hr |
| PT (prothrombin time) | 12.0 to 14.0 sec |
| PTT (partial thromboplastin time) | 35 to 45 sec |
| fibrinogen | 200 to 400 mg/dl |
| bleeding time | |
|    Duke method | 1 to 5 min |
|    Ivy method | Less than 5 min |
| coagulation time (Lee-White) | 5 to 15 min |
| Factor VIII | 50 to 150% of normal |

**Radioassay Thyroid Functions**

| | |
|---|---|
| $T_3$ uptake (tri-iodothyronine) | 25 to 38% |
| T4 (thyroxine) | 4.4 to 9.9 µg/dl |
| TSH (thyroid-stimulating hormone) | 0 to 7 microunits/ml |

**Serology**

| | |
|---|---|
| ANA (antinuclear antibody) | negative |
| CRP (C-reactive protein) | negative |
| RA latex (rheumatoid arthritis) | negative |
| RPR (rapid plasma reagin) | negative |
| VDRL (Venereal Disease Research Laboratory) | nonreactive |

**Urinalysis**

Routine

| | |
|---|---|
| color | yellow, straw, or colorless |
| sediment | clear or cloudy |
| sp. gr. (specific gravity) | 1.002 to 1.030 |
| pH | 4.5 to 8.0 (acid or alkaline) |
| nitrite | negative |
| protein or albumin | negative |

*Table continued on following page*

**Table 16–1. Normal Values for Laboratory Tests** *Continued*

Routine *continued*

| | |
|---|---|
| glucose | negative |
| acetone or ketones | negative |
| blood, occult | negative |
| bilirubin | 0.02 mg/dl |
| urobilinogen | 0.1 to 1.0 Ehrlich units/dl |

Microscopic

| | |
|---|---|
| RBC/hpf (red blood cells per high-powered field) | |
| WBC/hpf (white blood cells per high-powered field) | |
| epithelial cells/hpf | few or moderate |
| bacteria/lpf (low-powered field) | few or moderate |
| casts/lpf | negative |
| crystals/lpf | few |
| mucus | few or moderate |
| amorphous | few |

# 17

# LETTER

# FORMAT

## 17—1   ADDRESS

See Chapter 2, *Address Formats for Letters and Forms of Address.*

## 17—2 ATTENTION LINE

**_DO_**     type the attention line two spaces below the last line of the address, starting at the left margin. "Attention" may be spelled out in full caps or have only the first letter capitalized.

**_DO_**     use "Gentlemen" or "Dear Sir or Madam" as the salutation when using an attention line in a letter.

**_DO_**     insert the attention line in the inside address — between the name of the addressee and the street address or box number if using word processing equipment. This format allows easy generation of the envelope address.

**DON'T**   abbreviate the attention line or use any punctuation. It is optional to underline the word _Attention_.

## 17—3 BODY

**_DO_**     begin the body of the letter a double space from the salutation; use single-spacing. The first and subsequent lines are flush with the left margin unless indented paragraphs are used, in which case the first line of each paragraph is indented five spaces.

**_DO_**     double-space between paragraphs.

**_DO_**     leave at least two lines of the paragraph at the foot of one page and carry over at least two lines to the top of the next page.

**DON'T** divide a paragraph with only two or three lines between the bottom of one page and the top of the next.

## 17—4  COMPLIMENTARY CLOSE

See Figure 17–1.

***DO*** line up the complimentary close with the date and type it a double space below the last typed line. In a full block style letter, begin the closing at the left margin. The closing may be omitted in a simplified letter.

***DO*** capitalize only the first word in the complimentary close.

***DO*** use a comma after the complimentary close if a colon appears with the salutation (mixed punctuation).

Sincerely,          Sincerely yours,
Yours very truly,   Very truly yours,

***DO*** type the complimentary closing in its regular position, and type the informal phrase at the end of the last paragraph or as a separate paragraph with appropriate punctuation if using both a complimentary close and an informal closing phrase.

## 17—5  CONFIDENTIAL NOTATION

See Figure 17–1.

KARL ROBRECHT, M. D.　　　　　　ROBERT T. SACHS, M. D.
　Internal Medicine　　　　　　　　Physician and Surgeon

Gulf Medical Group
A Professional Corporation
800 Gulf Shore Boulevard
Naples, Florida 33940
Telephone 262-9976

| | | |
|---|---|---|
| Approximately 3 blank lines below letterhead | _____ | Date line |
| Second line below date line | _____ | Confidential or Personal notation |
| Fifth line below date line | _____ _____ _____ | Inside address |
| Double-space after last line of address | _____ : | Salutation |
| Double-space after salutation Single-spaced, with double space between paragraphs | _____ _____ _____ . _____ _____ _____ | Body |
| Double-space after last paragraph | _____ , | Complimentary close |
| 4 blank lines | | Signature area |
| | _____ | Typed signature line |
| | _____ | Title |
| Double-space | _____ | Reference initials |
| Double-space | _____ | Enclosure notation |
| Double-space | _____ | Distribution |
| Double-space | _____ | Postscript (P.S.) |

**Figure 17–1.** Business letter set-up mechanics showing modified block format and mixed punctuation. (See text for a description of each item illustrated.)

**_DO_**    type a personal notation on the second line below the date at the left margin. The notation may be typed in all-capital letters or in upper-case and lower-case letters that are underscored.

PERSONAL or <u>Personal</u>
CONFIDENTIAL or <u>Confidential</u>

## 17—6    CONTINUATION PAGES

**_DO_**    continue to the second page at the end of a paragraph whenever possible.

**_DO_**    leave at least two lines of the paragraph at the foot of one page and carry over at least two lines to the top of the next page.

**_DO_**    place headings one inch from the top of the page (See rule l7–18)

**DON'T**    type closer than one inch from the bottom of a page.

**DON'T**    divide a paragraph with only two or thee lines between the bottom of one page and the top of the next.

**DON'T**    divide the last word on the page.

---

---

**_DO_**     type a copy notation flush with the left margin a double space below the reference initials, mailing notation, or enclosure notation, whichever comes last. The abbreviation *cc* remains correct and popular. It used to mean "carbon copy" and now means "courtesy copy." Since most copies mailed out today are photocopies, some offices prefer to use the abbreviation *pc*.

    cc: Frank L. Naruse, M. D.
    c: Ruth Chriswell, Business Manager
    CC: Hodge W. Lloyd
    Copy: Carla P. Ralph, Buyer
    Copies:  Kristen A. Temple
                Anthony R. McClintock
    pc: John B. Smith, M. D.

**DON'T**     type a copy notation without a name following it.

**_DO_**     use a blind copy notation if the addressee is not intended to know that one or more persons are being sent a copy of the letter. This is noted on the file copy and the photocopy or carbon copy to the recipient in the upper left corner (starting at the left margin on the seventh line from the top) or typed on the second line below the last item in the letter (below the reference initials, enclosure notation, mailing notation, cc notation, or postscript).

    ***HANDY HINT.*** *When photocopying the original letter, type the blind copy notation on a removable adhesive note so the bcc notation will appear on your filed photocopy.*

    bcc Ms. Penelope R. Taylor (this is typed on the file copy and the copy to the recipient only)

**DO**      note on the file copy if enclosures are sent to other recipients of the correspondence. Usually, it is assumed that the enclosures accompany only the original letter.

     cc/enc: John L. Blake (received the letter and the enclosures)

**DON'T** make a copy notation on the original correspondence if the sender wishes a copy of the correspondence sent to a third party and does not wish the recipient of the original copy to know that this was done. See "Blind Copy Notation."

**DO**      use a check mark next to the name of the person for whom the copy is intended if copies are to be sent to several people.

     cc: Ms. Joan Cannon
         Ms. Harriet Newman   ✓

     (This letter was sent to Ms. Newman. The letter to be sent to Ms. Cannon would have a check mark by Ms. Cannon's name.)

## 17—8    DATE LINE

**DO**      type the date in keeping with the format of the letter and in line with the complimentary close and typed signature line. It is typed three lines below the letterhead (no closer but you may drop it farther down for a brief letter). The date used is the day the material was dictated, *not* the day it was transcribed.

**DO**      spell out the date in full in either the traditional or the military style.

December 22, 199x (traditional style)
22 December 199x (British and military style)

## 17—9 ENCLOSURE NOTATION

**DO**   type an enclosure notation flush with the left margin
if enclosing one or more items in a letter. The number
of enclosures should be noted if there is more than
one.

| Enc. | Enclosure | Check enclosed |
|------|-----------|----------------|
| Enc. 2 | 2 Enc. | 2 enclosures |
| Enclosed: | (1) History and physical | |
| | (2) Operative report | |
| | (3) Pathology report | |

*NOTE.   A one-page enclosure is not clipped or stapled to
a letter but is folded the same way as the letter and inserted into the last fold of the letter. An enclosure smaller
than the letter is stapled to the top of the letter in the upper left corner.*

## 17—10 FOLDING AND INSERTING

### No. 6-3/4 Envelope (6-1/2 x 3-5/8 Inches)

**DO**   bring the bottom edge of the sheet up to within one-
half inch of the top edge and fold. From the right
edge, fold over one third of the sheet, and crease.
From the left edge, fold the sheet so the left edge is
one-half inch from the right fold, and crease. Insert
the last creased edge into the envelope first.

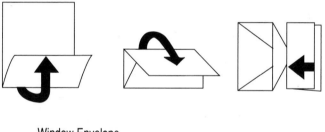

No. 10 Envelope (9-1/2 x 4-1/8 Inches)

___

**_DO_**  bring up the bottom third of the sheet, and crease. Fold down the upper third of the sheet so the top edge is a one-inch from the first fold, and crease. Insert the last creased edge into the envelope first.

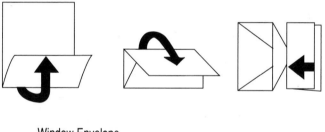

Window Envelope

___

**_DO_**  bring up the bottom third of the sheet and fold. Fold the top of the sheet _back_ to the first fold so that the inside address is on the outside, and crease. Insert the sheet so the address appears in the window.

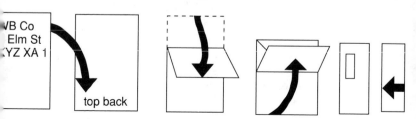

top back

## 17—11    FORMAT

**_DO_**    type all lines of the letter flush with the left margin in full block letter format. This includes date line, address, salutation, all lines of the body of the letter, complimentary close, and signature line (Fig. 17–2.)

**_DO_**    type the date line, complimentary close, and signature line just to the right of the middle of the page in modified block letter format (see Fig. 17–1.)

**_DO_**    indent paragraphs 5 spaces for modified block indented letter format.

**_DO_**    replace the salutation with an all-capital subject line and omit the complimentary close in simplified style. Begin all lines at the left margin. Type the signature line in all-capital letters on one line.

## 17—12    IN CARE OF

**_DO_**    use an "in care of" notation if a letter cannot be sent to the addressee's home or place of business and must be directed to a third person.

Ms. Margaret Shay
In care of Robert D. Hensley, M. D.

*or*

Ms. Margaret Shay
c/o Robert D. Hensley, M. D.

THORACIC SURGERY MEDICAL GROUP, INC.
Robert T. Steinway, M. D.
Stephen R. Clawson, M. D.
Christian M. Low, M. D.
Mary Sue Low, M. D.

504 Warford Drive                19098 Chatham Road
Syracuse, New York 13224         Syracuse, New York 13203
Telephone 466-4307               Telephone 279-2345

October 3, 199x

Matthew R. Bates, M. D.
7832 Johnson Avenue
Denver, CO 80241

Dear Dr. Bates:

RE: Leah Hamlyn

_____

_____

_____

_____  .

_____

_____

_____

_____

_____

_____

_____  .

_____

_____

_____  .

Sincerely yours,


Robert T. Steinway, President

mlo

cc: Eric T. Myhre

**Figure 17–2.** Letter illustrating full block format with closed punctuation and placement of reference or subject line.

## 17—13    INSIDE ADDRESS

See Chapter 2, *Address Formats for Letters and Forms of Address*

## 17—14    LETTERHEAD

**_DO_**    obtain approval from your employer before changing the letterhead, the type of printing, or the quality of the paper. The letterhead should contain the physician's name (or corporate name) and address, telephone number, medical specialty, and/or board membership.

## 17—15    LISTS

**_DO_**    type a list single-spaced with double spacing above and below the list. The list may be typed the full width of the letter or indented 5 spaces from each side margin. If an item in the list needs more than one line, leave a blank line between all items in the list. Align each line with the line above.

Dear Mrs. Hadley:

This is in reply to your letter concerning the results of your tests that were done here and by Dr. Galloway.

1) Intestinal symptoms, secondary to a
   lactose deficiency.
2) Generalized arteriosclerosis.
3) Mitral stenosis and insufficiency.
4) History of venous aneurysm.

You were seen on February 2, at which time you were having . . .

## 17—16    MAILING NOTATIONS

**DO**       type a mailing notation on the line below the reference initials or enclosure notation if a letter is to be delivered in a special way.

| | | |
|---|---|---|
| mtf | KMR:md | brt/lrt |
| Enc. 2 | By Federal Express | Enclosures 3 |
| Certified | cc Ms. Mary Evans | By messenger |

## 17—17    MARGINS

See Rule 17–28 on how to lengthen a letter.

**DO**       keep side margins of letters consistently in dimension and in keeping with the format style of the letter.

**DO**       leave a bottom margin of at least 6 lines (1 inch). However, if there is a second page to the letter, the bottom margin of the first page can be increased up to 12 lines (2 inches).

## 17—18    PAGE-ENDING CONSIDERATIONS

**DO**       leave a uniform margin of 6 to 12 lines at the bottom of each page of a letter (except the last page, which can be short).

**DON'T**   divide the last word on a page.

**DON'T** divide a paragraph that has only two or three lines. If a paragraph has four or more lines, leave at least two lines of the paragraph at the bottom of the previous page and carry over at least two lines to the continuation page.

**DON'T** use a continuation page to type only the complimentary close of a letter. The closing should be preceded by at least two lines of the body of the letter.

## 17—19    PARTS OF THE LETTER

See Figure 17–1 for the parts of the letter.

## 17—20    PERSONAL NOTATION

***DO*** use the words *personal* or *confidential* on the second line below the date, at the left margin, in upper-case letters or in underscored upper- and lower-case letters to indicate a personal notation (see Fig. 17–1).

PERSONAL or Personal
CONFIDENTIAL or Confidential

17—21    POSTSCRIPTS

**_DO_**    type a postscript (P.S., PS:, PS.) one double space below the last reference notation, flush with the left margin. If the paragraphs are indented, indent the first line of the postscript and bring the second and subsequent lines flush to the left margin. The P.S. can be an afterthought or a statement deliberately withheld from the body of the letter for emphasis or a restatement of an important thought, e.g., a phone number in a letter of application. If the afterthought reads in such a way that the letter looks poorly organized, insert the statement in the appropriate section of the letter. (Notice the spacing in the examples.)

P.S. By the way, I saw Flo Douglas in the elevator in St. Michaels Hospital the other day. She has certainly recovered nicely from her surgery. (afterthought)

P.S. Please do not hesitate to call on me if I can help you in any way. (emphasis)

**_DO_**    leave 2 spaces between the colon or period and the first word.

**_DO_**    type (P.P.S., PPS:, or PPS.) for an additional postscript, and double space down from the first postscript typed.

PS: Please do not hesitate to call on me if I can help you in any way.

PPS: I saw your patient Mrs. Erma Hamlyn at Cottage Hospital yesterday, and she seems to be much improved.

## 17—22 QUOTATIONS

See also Chapter 30, *Quotation Marks*.

**_DO_**  use single spacing and indent 5 spaces from each side margin for typing a quotation that is four or more typewritten lines. Double-space above and below the quotation. If the quotation is the beginning of an indented paragraph, indent the first word an additional 5 spaces.

**DON'T**  enclose the quotation in quote marks; the indention replaces the quotes.

## 17—23 REFERENCE INITIALS

**_DO_**  type the typist's initials alone in lower case, a double space below the typed signature line and type flush with the left margin. If the dictator wants his or her initials used, they should precede the initials of the typist. Otherwise, they may be omitted.

**_DO_**  type the dictator's, the signer's, and the typist's initials when the dictator differs from the person who signs the document.

mjp/arc/wpd                  or                  mjp:arc:wpd

Here, *mjp* stands for the dictator, *arc* stands for the signer, and *wpd* stands for the typist.

**DON'T** use humorous or confusing combinations of reference initials.

crc (rather than cc)
db (rather than dmb)
dg (rather than dog)

**DON'T** type your reference initials when you type a letter for your own signature.

## 17—24   REFERENCE OR SUBJECT LINE

*DO* type the patient's name a double space *after* the salutation in full block style (see Fig. 17–2).

*DO* type the patient's name in the blank space between the last line of the address and the salutation in modified block style. Align the patient's name with the date (Fig. 17–3).

---

THORACIC SURGERY MEDICAL GROUP, INC.
Robert T. Steinway, M. D.
Stephen R. Clawson, M. D.
Christian M. Low, M. D.
Mary Sue Low, M. D.

504 Warford Drive                                    19098 Chatham Road
Syracuse, New York 13224                  Syracuse, New York 13203
Telephone 466-4307                               Telephone 279-2345

                                                                      October 3, 199x

Matthew R. Bates, M. D.
7832 Johnson Avenue
Denver, CO 80241

                                                                      Re: Leah Hamlyn

Dear Dr. Bates:

---

**Figure 17–3.**   Letter showing modified block format with mixed punctuation at the salutation and placement of subject or reference line.

**DON'T**     place the reference or subject line in the wrong location, since dictators commonly dictate it out of place.

**DO**     use a subject line in place of the salutation in the simplified letter style. Begin the subject line on the third line below the inside address at the left margin, and type it in all-capital letters.

**DON'T**     use a term such as *Subject* to introduce the subject line in the simplified letter style.

**DO**     type a control reference notation two lines below the date or on the second line below any notation that follows the date.

When replying, refer to: VMT-501

**DO**     type the reference notation *Refer to:* or *RE.* Leave two spaces after the colon.

In reply to:  Z940 280 100 (file number)
Refer to:  Policy 90245 (insurance policy number)
RE:  Jennifer K. Hotta (name of patient)

**DO**     type your own reference notation before the addressee's reference notation when there are two reference notations. Type the addressee's reference notation on the second line below your reference notation. Double space between each notation.

When replying, refer to:  G-8043
Your reference:  BOX-Z-9

*NOTE. When replying to a letter that has a "refer to" notation, this may be typed in the subject line or below the date line.*

October 2, 199x
Refer to: Policy 90245

## 17—25    RETURN ADDRESS

**_DO_**    type a return address when using **plain paper**, listing the street address, city, state, ZIP code, and the date. The telephone number is optional. Allow a top margin of 1-1/2 to 2 inches. For modified block letter style, center the return address. For full block letter style, begin each line at the left margin.

479 East 53 Street, Apt. 45          or          Apartment 2B
New York, NY 10011-2706                             479 East 53 Street
October 4, 199x                                     New York, NY 10011-2706
                                                    (212) 458-0998
                                                    October 4, 199x

## 17—26    SALUTATION

See Chapter 2, *Address Formats for Letters and Forms of Address.*

**_DO_**    type the salutation a double space after the last line of the address using mixed (a colon) or open punctuation (no colon).

Dear Mr. Southerland:
Dear Mses. Ostrom and Allen: or Dear Ms. Ostrom
and Ms. Allen:
Dear Dr. Nappoi:
Dear Drs. Smith and Brown:   or    Dear Dr. Smith and
Dr. Brown:

When writing a firm:

Dear Sir or Madam:
Gentlemen:
Ladies:
Ladies and Gentlemen:

## 17—27    SIGNATURE LINE

___**DO**___       type the dictator's or writer's name exactly as it ap-
pears in the letterhead, four spaces after the complimentary close and aligned with it.

___**DO**___       type the dictator's or writer's official title when
preferred. If the title appears on the same line as the
name, it should be preceded by a comma. If the title is
typed on the line directly below the name, no comma
is needed.

Yours very truly,


Samuel R. Wong, M. D.
Chief-of-Staff


*or*


Sincerely,

Carla B. Black, M. D., Medical Director
(note the punctuation)

**_DO_**  identify an office employee's position in the firm and provide a courtesy title. The courtesy title (Miss, Ms., Mrs.) enables the correspondent to have a title to use in writing or telephoning. Enclose the courtesy title in parentheses.

(Ms.) Lynmarie Myhre, Secretary

(Mrs.) Elvira E. Gonsalves
Receptionist

(Miss) Paula de la Vera, CMA-A
Secretary to Dr. Bishop

**_DO_**  place two signature blocks side by side or one beneath the other when two people have to sign a letter.

## 17—28    SPACING

**_DO_**  type all letters single-spaced.

**_DO_**  lengthen a short letter by increasing the width of the margin.

## 17—29    SUBJECT LINE

See Rule 17–24, _Reference or Subject Line_ Figures 17–2 and 17–3.

## 17—30    TABLES

**_DO_**        center a table between the right and left margins when it occurs in the text of a letter.

**_DO_**        indent a minimum of 5 spaces from each side margin.

**_DO_**        allow from 2 to 6 spaces between columns.

**_DO_**        leave 1 to 3 blank lines above and below the table to set it apart from the rest of the text.

# 18

# Manuscripts

## 18—1   ABSTRACTS

**_DO_**  sequence the content of an abstract to follow that of the article. It should be double-spaced and contain the title, summary, and bibliographic information.

**_DO_**  use abbreviations and standard scientific symbols that are understood when used alone, such as pH and DNA.

The patient received HCT250. (incorrect)
The patient received hydrocortisone 250 mg. (correct)

The pH of the urine was 4.5. (correct)
The patient was discharged on aminophylline 200 mg q.i.d. (correct)

**DON'T**  use abbreviations that represent quantities with numerical values.

The patient received a u of insulin an hour. (incorrect)
The patient received one unit of insulin an hour. (correct)

**_DO_**  end the abstract with a complete bibliographic reference.

. . . intravascular coagulation played a significant role in the patient's death. In the second case prompt therapeutic maneuvers led to eventual recovery. (Wolfe BM, et al. Malignant hyperthermia of anesthesia. Am. J. Surg. Dec. 199x; 126:717–721.)

**DON'T**  list citations of references cited in the text of the article.

**DON'T**  include tables or figures.

## 18—2    BIBLIOGRAPHY

**_DO_**  list all works consulted in the preparation of the manuscript as well as all the papers that were cited in the notes. List authorship, title, edition, place of publication, publisher, date of publication, physical description (pages, illustrations, tables).

**_DO_**  arrange the bibliography in alphabetical order by the surnames of the authors (Fig. 18–1).

**_DO_**  put the bibliography on a separate page, titling the page with the word *bibliography* in all-capital letters and centered. Leave 2 blank lines and begin typing on line 16.

2 inches

BIBLIOGRAPHY

Item                                                    (Triple-space)

1. Follis, Joan L. and Marilyn T. Fordney, <u>Medical Office Procedures Worktext</u>, Syllabus, Ventura College, Ventura, California, 1977.

2. Franks, Richard, <u>Simplified Medical Dictionary</u>, Medical Economics/Delmar Publishers, Albany, New York, 1977.

3. Kinn, Mary E. and Eleanor Derge, <u>The Medical Assistant, Administrative and Clinical</u>, W. B. Saunders Company, Philadelphia, Pennsylvania, 1988.

4. Lessenberry, D. D. et al., <u>College Typewriting</u>, South-Western Publishing Company, Cincinnati, Ohio, 1975.

5. Lessenberry, D. D., S. J. Wanous, C. H. Duncan, and S. E. Warner, <u>College Typewriting</u>, Self-Paced Activities: An Individualized Approach, 9th edition, South-Western Publishing Company, Cincinnati, Ohio, 1976.

6. "Manuscript," <u>The World Book Encyclopedia</u>, 1970, XIII, p. 130.

7. Murphy, Lucie Spence, "Techniques On Writing the Medical Article," <u>Medical Record News</u>, American Medical Record Association, Chicago, Illinois, LIV, No. 6 (April, 1970), pp. 38–43.

8. <u>Oxnard Press Courier</u>, May 23, 1985, p. 15.

9. Swindle, Robert E., "Individualized Instruction in Business Communication," <u>Journal of Business Education</u>, Volume XL (May, 1973), pp. 335–336.

10. <u>United States Government Printing Office Style Manual</u>, Rev. ed., Washington, D. C., U. S. Government Printing Office, 1973.

The above bibliography shows reference styles for the following types of sources:

| | |
|---|---|
| 1. Unpublished manuscript | 6. Encyclopedia |
| 2. One-author book | 7. Bound volume of a periodical |
| 3. Two-author book | with page reference |
| 4. A book written by a number of authors | 8. Newspaper |
| | 9. Bound volume of a professional |
| 5. Book with subtitle and four authors | journal citing volume and page |
| | 10. Public document |

**Figure 18–1.** Illustration of a bibliography for a manuscript.

**_DO_**  use the same margins as the other pages in the body of the manuscript, and number the pages. (See Rules 18–11 and 18–12.)

**_DO_**  type each entry single-spaced at the left margin. Use double spacing if the manuscript is to be set in type. Indent the second line of each entry so the first word in each entry is easily visible.

**_DO_**  double-space between entries.

**_DO_**  use sentence-style capitalization.

**_DO_**  use periods at the end of each bibliographic entry, and use commas separating the elements within each entry, except for the title group. If the elements are not closely related, use a semicolon. Separate a title from a subtitle with a colon.

Sloane, Sheila B. and John L. Dusseau, <u>A Word Book in Pathology and Laboratory Medicine</u>, W. B. Saunders Company, Philadelphia, Pennsylvania, 1984.

**_NOTE._** *Bibliography format and punctuation can vary, depending on the publisher.*

## 18—3   BOOK REVIEW

**_DO_**  include the review heading (title), the text of the review, the author statement, and the author affiliation.

**_DO_** format the review heading with the same components as a bibliographic reference and, in addition, list the number of pages, illustrations, and tables, the price, the International Standard Book Number (ISBN), and where the book can be purchased (list an address). The ISBN number is given on the book's copyright page.

**_DO_** punctuate the review heading, following the same general principles used for punctuating bibliographic references.

**_DO_** list the author names exactly as they appear on the publication, and abbreviate authors' names only if that is how they appear on the publication.

A Word Book in Pathology and Laboratory Medicine. Sheila B. Sloane and John L. Dusseau. W. B. Saunders Company, Independence Square West, Philadelphia, Pennsylvania 19106-3399; 1984. 610 pages, 1 illustration, 14 tables. ISBN 0-7216-1099-4, $24.95.

## 18—4    CITATIONS

See *Endnotes*, Rule 18–6.

## 18—5    COPYRIGHT

**_DO_** place a copyright notice on the first page of the manuscript if the writer wishes to call attention to ownership of the material.

**_DO_** include the following elements in the copyright notice: copyright ©, current year, *by*, and the author's name.

## 18—6 ENDNOTES

Whenever words or ideas of a person other than the author appear in a manuscript, the author must provide the reader with the source of the words or ideas. Three common methods of doing this are by using (1) author/year citations, (2) endnotes, and (3) footnotes.

**_DO_** type the endnotes on a separate sheet. List them together at the end of each chapter or at the end of a complete report or manuscript. Type NOTES in all-capital letters, centered on line 13. Double-space and begin numbering and typing the first endnote. Single-space each endnote unless the manuscript is to be typeset, and in that case use double spacing to allow room for editing. Leave 1 blank line between endnotes. Indent the first line of each endnote 5 spaces. (See also *Footnotes*, Rule 18–7 and *Textnotes*, Rule 18–17.)

---

↓ 13

NOTES
↓3

    1. Sarah Augusta Taintor and Kate M. Munro, <u>The Secretary's Handbook.</u> The Macmillian Company, New York, New York, 1969, p. 435.

↓2

    2. Ibid. p. 180.[2]

---

**_NOTE._** *Endnote format and punctuation can vary, depending on the publisher.*

## 18—7    FOOTNOTES

**DO**    type a footnote that refers to a book. Include the footnote number, the author's name, the title (underscored), the edition (if not the first), the publisher, the place of publication, the year of publication, and the page reference. If the organization is more important than the contributors, list the organization's name (rather than the contributors) as author. (See also *Endnotes*, Rule 18–6 and *Textnotes*, Rule 18–17.)

**DO**    allow one-half inch for each footnote to be typed at the bottom of a page on which a reference is made.

**DO**    type an underscore 2 inches long at the bottom of the page to separate footnote material from the main text above. Type the underscore a double space below the last line of text, flush with the left margin.

**DO**    double-space below the underscore to type the first footnote.

**DO**    number and single-space each footnote and indent the first line five spaces. If the manuscript is to be typeset, use double spacing to allow for editing. Leave 1 blank line between each footnote.

-----

1. Sarah Augusta Taintor and Kate M. Munro, <u>The Secretary's Handbook</u>, The Macmillan Company, New York, New York, 1969, p. 435.
2. <u>Dorland's Illustrated Medical Dictionary</u>, 27th ed., W. B. Saunders Company, Philadelphia, Pennsylvania, 1988, p. 1888.

*NOTE. Footnote format and punctuation can vary, depending on the publisher.*

**DO** use the special Latin expressions in referring to a previously cited work to avoid repeating the original footnote in whole.

| Term | Meaning |
|---|---|
| c., cir. | about |
| ca., circa | about |
| cf. | compare |
| do. | ditto |
| e.g. | for example |
| et al. | and elsewhere or and others |
| et seq. | and the following |
| f. or ff. | following. Used after a page number to indicate that the next page or pages are also referred to. |
| ibid. | in the same place. Refers to a book, article, etc., cited in a reference immediately preceding. |
| i.e. | that is |
| l. | line |
| ll. | lines |
| loc. cit. | in the place cited. Refers to exactly the same place in a book, article, etc., cited in an earlier reference, but not the one immediately preceding. (For the latter reference you would use "ibid.") |
| ms or MS | manuscript |
| N.B. | note well |
| op. cit. | in the work cited. Refers to a book, article, etc., cited in a reference not immediately preceding. |
| sic | thus. Used to emphasize that an unlikely looking expression or spelling is really the one meant. |
| q.v. | which see |
| viz. | namely |

## 18—8    GALLEY PROOFS

**_DO_**    use formal proofreading marks to indicate corrections on galley proofs. The marks should appear at the site of the error in red pen as well as in right and/or left margins to draw the editor's eye to the line. (See also Chapter 28, *Proofreading and Revisions*.)

## 18—9    HEADINGS

See Figure 18—2.

**_DO_**    type in all-capital letters, centered on line 13. On the third line below the heading, begin typing the actual text.

**_DO_**    use three levels of text headings and subheadings (centered, side head, and run-in head). Centered headings may be typed in all-capital letters. Side headings begin flush with the left margin on a separate line and may be in all-capital letters or in capital and lower case letters that are underscored. Run-in or paragraph headings begin indented 5 spaces from the left margin and are immediately followed by text on the same line. Run-in headings should be typed in upper- and lower-case letters, underscored, and followed by a period. The text begins 2 spaces after the period.

1 or 1½
inch margin                          2 inches                          1 inch
                                                                       margin

Main Heading  TYPING A MEDICAL PROFESSIONAL REPORT
                                                    Triple-space
        This is your manuscript typing guide, which will help you
                                                    Double-space
prepare a manuscript for your physician. Always double-space

the body of the manuscript and indent five or ten spaces at the

beginning of each paragraph. Make a carbon copy of each page

and retain it for your records. The left margin should be 1 or

1½ inches, and the right margin should be 1 inch.


Title Page (Underline)
        A title page is not necessary for most manuscripts sub-
mitted for publication. If you need to type a page, refer to
Figure 18–4 for proper format.


Table of Contents (Underline)
        The table of contents is a list of headings of the major
parts of the manuscript. It is required by some, but not all,
publishers. When required, it is composed after the entire
manuscript has been completed so that correct page numbers
can be inserted. Notice that the entire table of contents has been
centered vertically in Figure 18–3.


                                1-inch
                                margin


**Figure 18–2.** Illustration of page one of a manuscript, showing format
and headings.

## 18—10    LEGENDS

**_DO_**     type on a separate sheet, double-spaced, and numbered to correspond with each figure in the manuscript. Place the author's name, the title of the manuscript, and the number of the figure on the back of each photograph or illustration.

## 18—11    MARGINS

See Figure 18–2.

**_DO_**     type double-spaced on 8-1/2 × 11 inch paper with 1-inch top, bottom, and side margins, except for a 2-inch top margin on the first page. If the manuscript is to be bound, the left margin should be 1-1/2 inches. Indent the first sentence of each paragraph five or ten spaces.

**_DO_**     try to keep the right margin as even as possible, and divide words according to proper word division guidelines. You may type two or three spaces beyond the desired right margin to avoid word division.

**DON'T**    have two consecutive end-of-line hyphenations.

**DON'T**    end a page with a hyphenated word.

# 18 Manuscripts

## 18—12    NUMBERING PAGES

**_DO_**   type page number 1 centered at the bottom of the page. Type the second and subsequent page numbers in the upper right-hand corner of the page.

## 18—13    PROOFREADING

**_DO_**   proofread the entire manuscript several times to check for clarity of meaning, spelling, punctuation, grammar, and other mechanics before it is submitted for publication.

**_DO_**   insert formal proofreading marks at the site of the error and in the right or left margins to call the editor's eye to the line in question. Marks should be made with a red pen.

## 18—14    SUMMARY

See Rule 18–1.

## 18—15    SYNOPSIS

See Rule 18–1

## 18—16    TABLE OF CONTENTS

**_DO_**     center the words _Contents_ or _Table of Contents_ in all-capital letters two inches from the top edge of the paper.

**_DO_**     list the major and minor headings with page numbers of the manuscript double- or single-spaced. Use leaders (a series of spaced dots) to guide the reader from the topic to its page number unless there are less than five entries (Fig. 18–3).

---

TABLE OF CONTENTS

TITLE PAGE . . . . . . . . . . . . . . . . . . . . . . . . . . . . . . . . . . . . . . .    0
TABLE OF CONTENTS . . . . . . . . . . . . . . . . . . . . . . . . . . . .    0
BODY OF MANUSCRIPT. . . . . . . . . . . . . . . . . . . . . . . . . .    0
Margins . . . . . . . . . . . . . . . . . . . . . . . . . . . . . . . . . . . . . . . . .    0
Headings . . . . . . . . . . . . . . . . . . . . . . . . . . . . . . . . . . . . . . . .    0
Footnotes . . . . . . . . . . . . . . . . . . . . . . . . . . . . . . . . . . . . . . . .    0
BIBLIOGRAPHY . . . . . . . . . . . . . . . . . . . . . . . . . . . . . . . .__0

3 spaces

---

**Figure 18–3.**    Illustration of a table of contents for a manuscript.

**_DO_**     include supplemental parts of the manuscript (appendix, bibliography, index), with their page numbers.

# 18 Manuscripts

**DO**  type the textnote directly below the statement referred to and separated by two solid lines. Number and indent each textnote five spaces. Textnotes may be single- or double-spaced. (See also *Endnotes*, Rule 18–6, and *Footnotes*, Rule 18–7.)

A manuscript submitted to an editor, publisher, or printer should be carefully and attractively typed.[1]

---

1. Sarah Augusta Taintor and Kate M. Munro, <u>The Secretary's Handbook,</u> The Macmillan Company, New York, New York, 1969, p. 435.

---

**NOTE.** *Textnote format and punctuation can vary, depending on the publisher.*

## 18—18    TITLE PAGE

***DO***   include the title of the report in all-capital letters, as well as the name and title of the author, the group or organization of the intended reader, and the date. It is optional to precede the name with the words *prepared for* or *submitted by* (Fig. 18–4).

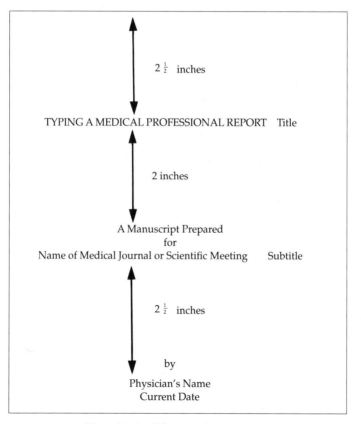

**Figure 18–4.**   Title page of a manuscript.

# 19

# MEDICAL

# REPORTS

## INTRODUCTION

Use the formats and standard outlines preferred in your locality and/or hospital facility. Appearance and ease of readability are important factors.

# 19 MEDICAL REPORTS

## 19—1 AUTOPSY PROTOCOLS

**DO**     refer to your County Coroner's Office and State Board of Medical Examiners for the legal requirements when typing and reporting autopsy protocols, since only general guidelines are stated here.

**DO**     type an autopsy in one of the five pathology forms: the narrative (in story form), the numerical (by the numbers), the pictorial (hand drawings or anatomic forms), protocols based on sentence completion and multiple-choice selection, or problem-oriented protocols (a supplement to the Problem-Oriented Medical Record System) (Fig. 19–1).

**DO**     spell out abbreviations or keep them to a minimum because clarity is the essential element in an autopsy. Interpretation of typed material must be accurate.

**DO**     use military time if required by state law when documenting the time a body is brought in for autopsy.

1400 hours

**DO**     use the wording *found over the date of January 1, 199x* if a person was last seen before midnight. If a person was last seen after midnight, state *found over the hour of 9:00 a.m. or 0900*.

**Figure 19–1.** Hospital Autopsy Protocol, typed in narrative report form and in indented format with no variations.

---

College Hospital
4567 Broad Avenue
Woodland Hills, XY 12345

AUTOPSY REPORT

Silverman, Patricia M.
College Hospital
June 20, 199x

This is an autopsy report on a prematurely born female infant weighing 2 pounds 12 ounces. The body measures 15.25 inches in length. The body has not been embalmed prior to this examination.

EXTERNAL EXAMINATION:  The head, neck, and chest are symmetrical. The abdomen is soft. The external genitalia are normal female. The extremities are symmetrical and show no evidence of developmental abnormality.

INTERNAL EXAMINATION:

ABDOMINAL CAVITY:  The abdominal cavity is opened and the liver is enlarged, extending 4 cm below the costal margin in the right midclavicular line. The spleen appears enlarged. The intestinal coils are freely dispersed and contain gaseous fluid. All other organs are in normal position.

PLEURAL CAVITIES:  The pleural cavities are opened, revealing the left lung to be collapsed and lying in the left pleural cavity. The right lung is partially expanded, and the pleura is smooth and glistening in both pleural cavities.

MEDIASTINUM:  The mediastinum contains a moderate amount of thymic tissue.

PERICARDIAL SAC:  The pericardial sac is opened, containing a few cubic centimeters of serous fluid. The heart is normal in position and appears to be average in size.

HEART:  The heart weighs approximately 10 grams. Thorough search of the heart

(continued)

---

*Illustration continued on next page*

Patricia M. Silverman
Page 2
June 20, 199x

<u>INTERNAL EXAMINATION</u>: (continued)

fails to show any evidence of congenital abnormality. The foramen ovale has a thin membrane over the surface. The ductus arteriosus is noted and patent. There is no septal ventricular defect. All valves are competent. There is no rotation of the heart. The pulmonary artery is noted and appears normal. A few subendocardial and subepicardial petechiae and ecchymoses are noted.

LUNGS:                           The lungs together weigh 33 grams. The left lung and the right lung sink in water, then slowly rise to the surface. The lungs are subcrepitant and atelectatic. This is particularly noted in the left lung. The bronchi contain a small amount of frothy mucus. The cut surfaces of the lungs are beefy and atelectatic. There are no cysts or tumors. The findings are consistent with hyaline membrane disease and pulmonary atelectasis.

LIVER:                           The liver weighs approximately 75 grams. The liver appears enlarged and is reddish-brown and soft. The cut surface is reddish-brown and soft. There is no gross evidence of bile duct blockage. The gallbladder, cystic duct, and common bile duct are not remarkable.

PANCREAS:                        The pancreas appears average in size, weighing approximately 1.5 grams. The pancreas is yellowish-white and soft on the cut surface. There is no gross evidence of cystic disease.

SPLEEN:                          The spleen weighs approximately 4 grams and is bluish-purple. The spleen on cut surface is reddish-brown and soft.

ADRENAL GLANDS:                  The adrenal glands together weigh approximately 4.5 grams. The adrenal glands are soft and tan and the cortical portion is distinct from the medullary portion. There is no gross evidence of hemorrhage, cysts, or tumors. Both adrenals are similar.

(continued)

Patricia M. Silverman
Page 3
June 20, 199x

<u>INTERNAL EXAMINATION</u>: (continued)

KIDNEYS: The kidneys weigh together approximately 13 grams. The capsule strips with ease, leaving a faint fetal lobulation and a reddish-brown soft surface. The cut surface shows the cortex and medulla, both of which are distinct and in average proportions. The parenchyma is reddish-brown, moist, and soft. Both kidneys are similar in appearance and consistency. The ureters are not remarkable.

URINARY BLADDER, UTERUS, TUBES AND OVARIES: These organs are grossly not remarkable.

GASTROINTESTINAL TRACT: The esophagus, as well as the stomach, is examined. There is no evidence of reduplication, ulcer, or tumor. The small and large bowels are not remarkable.

BRAIN: The brain weighs approximately 230 grams. The brain is slightly edematous. A few petechiae are observed. On sectioning the brain anterior to posterior, the brain tissue is soft and somewhat edematous. The fluid in the ventricles is clear and watery. The cerebellum and cerebrum are symmetrical and grossly not remarkable. There is no gross evidence of hemorrhage or tumor.

SKELETAL SYSTEM: Not remarkable.

<u>GROSS ANATOMIC</u> <u>DIAGNOSES</u>:
1) Prematurity, 2 pounds 12 ounces.
2) Pulmonary atelectasis.
3) Hyaline membrane disease.

Chief Pathologist _____

Stephen M. Choi, M.D.

mtf
D: 6-20-9x
T: 6-21-9x

**_DO_**     abbreviate when typing metric terms.

0.5 cm     200 ml     3 × 3 mm     100 cc

**NOTE.** *Regarding weights of organs, many facilities prefer that transcriptionists spell out the word grams in hospital autopsy reports and forensic autopsy reports. When abbreviated, it is typed either* gm *or* g.

The heart weighs 330 grams.

**_DO_**     spell out pounds and inches.

The body weighs 160 pounds, and the body length is 65 inches.

**_DO_**     spell out all words when typing the body temperature.

88 degrees Fahrenheit

**_DO_**     spell out and put in parentheses numbers indicating how much or how many whenever clarity needs to be emphasized.

two (2) stab wounds

**_DO_**     use quote marks when indicating a marking on the body.

A superficial "V" shaped suture wound is present on the left cheek.

A tattoo device of the words "J. J. Tramp" appears on the left knee.

**DON'T** use quote marks to indicate inches.

22" (incorrect)
22 inches (correct)

*DO* in a *hospital autopsy protocol* include the following:

Clinical History (a brief resume of the patient's medical history and course in the hospital prior to demise)
Pathologic Diagnosis (at autopsy)
External Examination
Macroscopic Examination
Internal Examination
Gross Findings (visual examination of the organs of the body before any tissues are removed for preparation and examination)
Microscopic Examination (an examination of the particular organs through the microscope)
Epicrisis or Final Pathologic Diagnosis (critical analysis or actual finding or discussion of the cause of disease after its termination).
Report of Final Summary or Discussion
Signature of pathologist

*DO* include the following in a *forensic pathology autopsy protocol*:

External Description
Evidence of Injury (external and internal)
Systems and Organs (cavities and organs)
Special Dissections and Examinations
Brain (and other organs) After Fixation
Microscopic Examination
Findings (diagnoses), Factual and Interpretative
Opinion (conclusion), Interpretative and Opinion
Signature of medical examiner/pathologist

> **NOTE.** *Forensic dentists describe bite marks by size, shape, and location. They swab for saliva to determine blood type, make impressions or molds of the bite mark, and photograph and make impressions of the suspect's dentition.*

**_DO_**    type both reference initials, as well as your own, when two medical examiners are involved.

MB:DVW:mtf

## 19—2    COMPUTER FORMAT

**_DO_**    use full block report style to reduce the number and complexity of machine manipulations required. This will save time and reduce errors.

**_DO_**    use single, double, or quadruple spacing when keying a report.

**DON'T**    use triple-space conventions in documents, as this consumes time and invites spacing errors since multiple key codes must be inserted.

**_DO_**    type sub- and superscripts on one line to save time or if your software and/or equipment does not have capabilities of printing small numbers above or below the line (see Rule 22–24).

V-4, L4-5, vitamin B12, $CO_2$, O2, A2, P2, V1 through V6

## 19—3    CONSULTATION REPORTS

**_DO_**        type in letter form or report form, single-spaced, with content similar to a history and physical medical report. Headings may or may not be included. Send to the attending physician who requested the consultation. The report should be signed by the examining physician (Fig. 19–2). See also Chapter 14, _History and Physical Format_.

## 19—4    CONTINUATION SHEETS

**_DO_**        type headings for page 2 and subsequent pages using the format preferred by your employer and/or hospital facility. This would include the patient's name, medical record number, page number, and other optional statistical information (name of attending physician).

**_DO_**        type flush with the left margin or use a horizontal format.

Maria J. Valdez
#6893
Page 2

_or_

Maria J. Valdez          #6893          Page 2

**_DO_**        type _continued_ on the bottom of all incomplete sheets, beginning with the first page, when the report includes more than one page.

**Figure 19–2.** Consultation Report generated from a medical clinic, typed in letter form and in modified block format with indented paragraphs and mixed punctuation.

REDLANDS CLINIC
6000 Main Street
Woodland Hills, XY 12345

July 8, 199x

Katherine M. Fukuda, M. D.
5409 Center Street
Woodland Hills, XY 12345

Dear Dr. Fukuda:

RE: Philip B. Osterman

This 78-year-old gentleman referred by Dr. Fukuda was also seen by Dr. Mason at the Redlands Clinic. He has been seen in the past by Dr. Klugman.

The patient developed a lesion in the concha of the left external ear. Recent biopsy confirmed this as being a squamous cell carcinoma. The patient has had a few other skin cancers.

Of most significant past history is the fact that this patient has a leukemia that has been treated in standard fashion by Dr. Klugman. The patient was then transferred to the Redlands Clinic and by some experimental protocol which, I guess, includes some sort of lymphocyte electrophoresis, has been placed into a remission. He is not currently on any antileukemia drugs and has responded extremely well to his medical management.

On examination the patient is healthy in general appearance. There is a 1.5 cm lesion in the concha of the ear, which is seen well on photograph of the left external ear. There are numerous soft lymph nodes in both sides of the neck, which I presume are related to his leukemia.

Diagnosis: Squamous cell carcinoma, relatively superficial, involving the skin of the left external ear.

The plan of treatment is as follows: 4500 rad, 15 treatment sessions, using 100 kV radiation.

The reason for treatment, expected acute reaction, and remote possbility of complication was discussed with this patient at some length, and he accepted therapy as outlined.

Sincerely,

David M. Packer, M. D.

mtf

**DON'T**     carry just one line of a medical report to a continuation sheet.

**DON'T**     carry only the signature line to a continuation sheet.

## 19—5    CORRECTIONS

***DO***     retain the original transcript when corrections necessitate retyping a medical report in hospital transcription. The physician should insert omitted words, correct all errors, and initial each correction directly on the original transcript. On the second draft, type *corrected for typing errors*. The physician should sign both copies, and they should be stapled together.

## 19—6    DATES

***DO***     use the date the material was dictated, not the day it was transcribed, in hospital generated reports.

***DO***     spell out the date in full in either the traditional or the military style.

     November 14, 199x (traditional)
     22 December 199x (British and military)

***DO***     type the dates of dictation and transcription at the end of the hospital medical report on two lines below the reference initials.

     mtf:jf
     D: 11-24-9x
     T: 11-25-9x

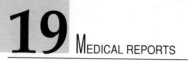

---

## 19—7    DIAGNOSIS

---

**_DO_**       spell out any terms dictated as abbreviations in the diagnosis portion of any medical report.

DIAGNOSIS: ASHD (incorrect)
DIAGNOSIS: Arteriosclerotic heart disease (correct)

**_DO_**       use numbering if dictated; it is optional if not dictated.

DIAGNOSES:  Gastritis.
                        Pancreatitis.

_or_

DIAGNOSES:
1.  Gastritis.
2.  Pancreatitis.

## 19—8    DISCHARGE SUMMARIES, CLINICAL RESUMES, or FINAL PROGRESS NOTES (Fig. 19–3)

---

**Figure 19–3.** A hospital Discharge Summary, typed in report form and full block format. The absence of a letterhead and the final two notations on the left side of the page indicate that this report was prepared by a hospital transcriptionist.

Silverman, Elaine J.
90-32-11
July 15, 199x

DISCHARGE SUMMARY

ADMISSION DATE: June 14, 199x
DISCHARGE DATE: July 15, 199x

HISTORY OF PRESENT ILLNESS:
This 19-year-old black female, nulligravida, was admitted to the hospital on June 14, 199x with fever of 102°, left lower quadrant pain, vaginal discharge, constipation, and a tender left adnexal mass. Her past history and family history were unremarkable. Present pain had started 2 to 3 weeks prior (starting on May 30, 199x) and lasted for 6 days. She had taken contraceptive pills in the past but had stopped because she was not sexually active.

PHYSICAL EXAMINATION:
She appeared well developed and well nourished, and in mild distress. The only positive physical findings were limited to the abdomen and pelvis. Her abdomen was mildly distended, and it was tender, especially in the left lower quadrant. At pelvic examination her cervix was tender on motion, and the uterus was of normal size, retroverted, and somewhat fixed. There was a tender cystic mass about 4–5 cm in the left adnexa. Rectal examination was negative.

ADMITTING DIAGNOSIS:
1. Probable pelvic inflammatory disease (PID).
2. Rule out ectopic pregnancy.

LABORATORY DATA ON ADMISSION:
Hb 8.8, Hct 26.5, WBC 8,100 with 80 segs and 18 lymphs. Sedimentation rate 100 mm in one hour. Sickle cell prep + (turned out to be a trait). Urinalysis normal. Electrolytes normal. SMA-12 normal. Chest x-ray negative, 2-hour UCG negative.

(continued)

*Illustration continued on next page*

Page 2
Elaine J. Silverman
Hospital No. 90-32-11

HOSPITAL COURSE AND TREATMENT:
Initially, she was given cephalothin 2 gm IV q6h, and
kanamycin 0.5 gm IM b.i.d. Over the next 2 days the patient's
condition improved. Her pain decreased, and her temperature
came down to normal in the morning and spiked to 101° in the
evening. Repeat CBC showed Hb 7.8, Hct 23.5. The pregnancy
test was negative. On the second night following admission, her
temperature spiked to 104°. The patient was started on anti-
tuberculosis treatment, consisting of isoniazid 300 mg/day,
ethambutol 600 mg b.i.d., and rifampin 600 mg daily. She became afebrile on the sixth postoperative day and was discharged on July 15, 199x, in good condition. She will be seen in
the office in one week.

SURGICAL PROCEDURES:
Biopsy of omentum for frozen section; culture specimens.

DISCHARGE DIAGNOSIS:
Genital tuberculosis.

Surgeon _____
Harold B. Cooper, M.D.

mtf
D: 7-15-9x
T: 7-16-9x

**DO**  type single-spaced with main headings, whether dictated or not, and insert those subheadings as dictated:

> Admission Date
> Discharge Date
> History of Present Illness
> Physical Examination
> Admitting Diagnosis
> Laboratory and/or X-ray Data on Admission
> Hospital Course and Treatment
> Surgical Procedures
> Consultations
> Discharge Diagnosis
> Condition of the Patient on Discharge (medications on discharge, instructions for continuing care, therapy, and follow-up postoperative office visit date)

> **NOTE.** *In the case of death, a summary statement should be added to the record either as a final progress note or as a separate resume. This final note should give the reason for admission, the findings and course of illness in the hospital, and events leading to death.*

**DO**  send a copy of the discharge summary to any known medical practitioner and/or medical facility responsible for follow-up care of the patient if authorized in writing by the patient or his/her legally qualified representative.

## 19—9  FORMAT STYLES

See Rule 14–3, *Format Styles*, and Rule 19–2, *Computer Format.*

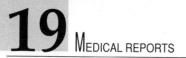

## 19—10   HEADINGS

**_DO_**    type major headings in all capitals followed by a colon. Place major headings on a line alone and underline, depending on your format style choice. (See Rule 14–3, *Format Styles*.) If the dictator moves in and out of paragraphs and does not dictate complete paragraphs, omit or add headings, depending on your employer's preference.

## 19—11   HISTORY AND PHYSICAL FORMAT

See Chapter 14, *History and Physical Format*.

## 19—12   MARGINS

**_DO_**    use one-half inch to three-quarter inch right and left and bottom margins.

## 19—13   MEDICOLEGAL REPORTS

**_DO_**    type on the physician's letterhead stationery in letter format, with or without headings and/or subheadings, a detailed document that includes the following information (Fig. 19–4):

**Figure 19–4.** Medicolegal Report generated from a medical office, typed in report form and in indented format with no underlining and mixed punctuation.

---

CLARENCE F. STONES, M. D.
3700 OCEAN DRIVE
WOODLAND HILLS, XY 12345

October 20, 199x

Aetna Casualty and Surety Company
3200 Roosevelt Boulevard
Woodland Hills, XY 12345

                Re:  Injured - Howard P. Winston
                     Date of Injury - July 27, 199x
                     Employer - College Chemistry Co.
                     Case No. - 450-33-0821

Gentlemen:

EXAMINATION AND REPORT

HISTORY:            This 43-year-old white male was working with a
                     chemical pump. It slipped and fell forward. He over-
corrected and fell. The pump fell on the patient, striking him in the oc-
cipital area. The approximate weight of the pump was 325 lb and was
rolled off by a friend. He was knocked unconscious. He attended a meeting the following day in San Mateo. The pain occurred a day later in San
Mateo. Three days later the pain was intense in the right shoulder and elbow. He went to Dr. John Garrett for physiotherapy. The left side then
began to give him trouble also. He had a pressure type of pain in the left
elbow, which was relieved by codeine. He entered the College Hospital in
Woodland Hills under Dr. Garrett's service. The right leg, and later the
right thigh, began getting numb. A myelogram was followed by fusion at
C5–6 and C6–7. He wore a brace for six months. He still has right
shoulder pain, and neck pain with radiation into the right thumb and
right mastoid. In June, 199x, he was admitted to the Community Hospital
in Ventura, California. The left eye began drooping, and there was no
pupil dilatation. He was improved one week later. A myelogram and
brain scan were performed. There was pain on the left side, with pain
into the rectum with spasms. He states that he fell several times. The surgery was postponed because of the eyes and the sudden loss of equi-
librium.

FAMILY HISTORY:   The father died of burns in a fire in 1940. The
                        mother died of kidney disease at age 82. He has
two brothers and one sister, living and well. He is widowed. His wife had

(continued)

---

Howard P. Winston
Page 2
October 20, 199x

FAMILY HISTORY: (continued)

cancer of the uterus. He has four children, alive and well. There is no history of diabetes and no accidents.

ALLERGIES: <u>Penicillin</u> and <u>tetanus</u>.

PHYSICAL
EXAMINATION: Blood pressure 122/78; pulse 84 and regular.

GENERAL: The patient is cooperative and oriented to time and place.

HEENT: Head: Normal size and shape; no facial asymmetry. He shows no evidence of elevated intracranial pressure. Extraocular muscles intact. Pupils are equal and react briskly to light. At first one gets the impression that Horner's syndrome might be present on the left side because of inconstant ptosis of the right eyelid, but it is not truly present.

NEUROLOGIC The patient walks with sparing of the left leg.
EXAM: There is no true paralysis present.

REFLEXES: The right biceps and triceps are slightly reduced on the left side, but present.

SENSORY: There is evidence of patchy hyperesthesia in the right upper extremity but following no particular dermatomal pattern.

CEREBELLAR Intact. Lower cranial nerves within normal limits.
FUNCTION: There were no pathologic reflexes elicited.
The remaining exam was deferred.

OPINION AND The patient continues to have slight dysfunction
COMMENT: principally in the left lower extremity and right upper extremity. It would seem to me that the pupillary abnormality, which he experienced in June of 199x, merits some investigation, including arteriography. For his cervical disk problems, I would think that conservative treatment is warranted.

Very truly yours,

Clarence F. Stones, M.D.

mtf

Patient's name
Date of the accident or injury
History of the accident, injury, or illness
Present complaint(s)
Past history and pre-existing conditions
Physical findings on examination
Laboratory and/or x-ray findings
Diagnosis
Prescribed therapy
Disability
Prognosis

## 19—14  NUMBERING

***DO***    be consistent in using Arabic numerals to number vertically or horizontally all or none of the entries when typing if the dictator numbers some but not all terms in a series. Capitalize the first letter of each numbered entry and place a period at the end of each statement.

        DISCHARGE DIAGNOSES: 1. Tube pregnancy delivered by repeat cesarean section.
                                2. Postoperative lower segment placental bed sinus hemorrhage of the uterus.

        ADMITTING DIAGNOSES: (1) Left pleural effusion, (2) Left otitis media, (3) Procaine-induced lupus-like syndrome.

        DIAGNOSES:
1. Diabetes out of control.
2. Acute alcohol intoxication.
3. Peripheral neuropathy.
4. History of thyroidectomy.

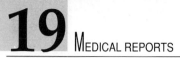

# 19 Medical Reports

## 19—15 OPERATIVE REPORTS (Fig. 19–5)

See also Rule 22–25 on how to type suture materials.

***DO***    type on a printed form or on plain paper the name of the patient, the room number, the hospital number, the surgeon's name, the assistant surgeon's name, and the date of the operation.

***DO***    type single-spaced with main headings, whether dictated or not, and insert those subheadings (anesthesia, incision, sponge count, closure, and so forth) as dictated. Include the following headings in the report:

> Preoperative Diagnosis
> Postoperative Diagnosis
> Operation Performed
>> Many hospitals break down the operative description into three sections: (1) positioning, prepping, and draping and opening the incision; (2) the internal operation; and (3) the closing.
>
> Procedure or Findings
> Signature of the surgeon

> ***NOTE.*** *Some hospital policies require that if there is a dictation/transcription and/or filing delay, a comprehensive operative progress note must be entered in the medical record immediately after surgery in order to provide pertinent information for other physicians who may be attending the patient.*

**Figure 19–5.** A hospital Operative Report, typed in report form and in indented format with the body of the report done in one or two large paragraphs.

---

COLLEGE HOSPITAL
4567 Broad Avenue
Woodland Hills, XY 12345

Patient: Elaine J. Silverman               Date: June 20, 199x

Hospital No.: 90-32-11                     Room No.: 1308

OPERATIVE REPORT

PREOPERATIVE DIAGNOSES:
1. Menorrhagia.
2. Chronic pelvic inflammatory disease.
3. Perineal relaxation.

POSTOPERATIVE DIAGNOSES:
1. Menorrhagia.
2. Chronic pelvic inflammatory disease.
3. Perineal relaxation.

OPERATIONS:
1. Total abdominal hysterectomy.
2. Lysis of pelvic adhesions.
3. Bilateral salpingo-oophorectomy.
4. Appendectomy.
5. Posterior colpoplasty.

PROCEDURE:                 Under general anesthesia, the patient was prepared and draped for abdominal operation. The abdomen was opened through a Pfannenstiel incision, and examination of the upper abdomen was entirely normal. Examination of the pelvis revealed an enlarged uterus. The uterus was three degrees retroverted and adhered to the cul-de-sac. Both tubes and ovaries were involved in an inflammatory mass, with extensive ad-

(continued)

---

*Illustration continued on next page*

Elaine J. Silverman          Page 2          Hospital No. 90-32-11

PROCEDURE: (continued)

hesions to the lateral pelvic wall on both sides. The tubes revealed evidence of chronic pelvic inflammatory disease. The omentum was also attached to the fundus and to the left adnexa. The omentum was dissected by means of blunt and sharp dissection; the dissection was carried to each adnexa, freeing both tubes and ovaries by means of blunt and sharp dissection. The uterus was found to be approximately two times enlarged, after freeing all the adhesions. The uterovesical fold of peritoneum was then incised in an elliptical manner; bladder was dissected off the lower uterine segment. The round ligament, infundibulopelvic ligament on each side was identified, clamped, cut, and ligated. The uterine artery on each side was clamped, cut, and doubly ligated. Paracervical fascia was developed. Heaney clamps were placed on the cardinal ligaments, the cardinal ligaments cut, and pedicles ligated. The vagina was circumscribed; the uterus, both tubes and ovaries were removed from the operative field. The cardinal ligaments were then sutured into the lateral angles of the vagina by means of interrupted sutures; the vagina was then closed with continuous over-and-over stitch. The paracervical fascia was sutured into place with interrupted figure-of-eight sutures; the lateral suture incorporated the stumps of the uterine arteries; the pelvis was then reperitonealized with continuous length of GI 2–0 atraumatic suture.

Appendix was identified, and appendectomy was done in the usual manner. The appendiceal stump was cauterized with phenol and neutralized with alcohol. Re-examination of the pelvis at this time revealed all bleeding well controlled. The abdominal wall was then closed in layers, and the skin was approximated with camelback clips. During the procedure, the patient received one unit of blood. Patient was then prepared for vaginal surgery.

Patient was placed in lithotomy position, prepared and draped. Posterior colpoplasty was begun, for repair of rectocele and perineal relaxation. The posterior vaginal mucosa was dissected

(continued)

---

Elaine J. Silverman　　　　Page 3　　　　Hospital No. 90-32-11

PROCEDURE: (continued)

from the perirectal fascia; the excess posterior vaginal mucosa was excised and perirectal fascia was brought together with continuous interlocking suture of 0 chromic. The posterior vaginal mucosa was closed with continuous interlocking suture of 0 chromic. Perineal body was closed with subcutaneous, subcuticular stitch. There was a correct sponge count. The patient withstood the operation well. Patient left the operating room in good condition.

Surgeon _____
　　　　　　Harold B. Cooper, M.D.


mtf
D: 6-20-9x
T: 6-22-9x

---

## 19—16　OUTLINE

For outline rules, see *Autopsy Protocols, Consultation Reports, Discharge Summaries, Clinical Resumes, or Final Progress Notes, Medicolegal Reports, Operative Reports, Pathology Reports,* and *Radiology Reports* in this chapter.

See Chapter 14, *History and Physical Format* for history and physical outlines.

## 19—17　PATHOLOGY REPORTS (Fig. 19–6)

See also Rule 19–1, *Autopsy Protocols*.

**_DO_**　　　　type on a printed form or on plain paper the pathology identification number, the name of the patient, the room number, the hospital number, and the date of the operation.

**Figure 19–6.**  A Pathology Report generated in a hospital, typed in report form and in modified block format with no variations.

---

College Hospital
4567 Broad Avenue
Woodland Hills, XY 12345

PATHOLOGY REPORT

| | | |
|---|---|---|
| Date: | June 18, 199x | Pathology No. 430211 |
| Patient: | Elaine J. Silverman | Room No. 1308 |
| Physician: | Harold B. Cooper, M.D. | Hospital No. 90-32-11 |
| Specimen Submitted: | Tissue from left forearm | |

GROSS DESCRIPTION:

Specimen is an elliptical segment of cutaneous tissue which exhibits hemorrhage in the subcutaneous adipose tissue of recent origin. The specimen measures $10 \times 7 \times 5$ mm. There is a cylindrical shaped segment of gray, moderately firm material measuring $6 \times 1$ cm. This is sharp and consistent with a foreign body. The cutaneous and subcutaneous tissue is bisected and is totally embedded.

MICROSCOPIC DESCRIPTION:

Examination reveals a well-demarcated dermal neoplasm. There are clear cells and squamous cells in this well-demarcated area associated with ductal structures resembling sweat gland ducts. Areas of hyalinization and fibrosis are also present. Recent areas of hemorrhage are associated with the neoplasm. Cystic spaces within the neoplasm are present. Individual nuclei are found, and mitotic figures are not seen.

DIAGNOSIS:

Tissue from left forearm:  ECCRINE SPIRADENOMA, BENIGN.

Pathologist  _____
Carl B. Skinner, M.D.

mtf
D:  6-18-9x
T:  6-20-9x

---

**_DO_**    type single-spaced with main headings whether dictated or not.

> Gross or Macroscopic Description
> Microscopic Description
> Comment
> Recommendation
> Conclusion(s) and/or Diagnosis
> Signature of the pathologist

**_DO_**    type in all capitals and/or underline the section of the pathology report detailing benign or malignant lesions.

> A frozen section consultation at the time of surgery was delivered as NO EVIDENCE OF MALIGNANCY on frozen section, to await permanent section for final diagnosis.

## 19—18    RADIOLOGY REPORTS (Fig. 19–7)

**_DO_**    type on a printed form or on plain paper the name of the patient, the name of the attending physician, the radiology identification number, the patient's age, the date, and the type of examination. In addition, in a hospital case, type in the room number and the hospital number.

**_DO_**    type single-spaced with main headings, whether dictated or not.

> Name of the x-ray, x-ray examination, scan, xeroradiography, thermography, nuclear magnetic resonance, ultrasound, and so forth.
> Findings or interpretation
> Impression or diagnosis
> Conclusion
> Recommendations
> Signature of the radiologist

**Figure 19–7.** A hospital Radiology Report, typed in report form and in modified block format with no variations.

---

RADIOLOGY REPORT

| | | | |
|---|---|---|---|
| Examination Date: | June 14, 199x | Patient: | Elaine J. Silverman |
| Date Reported: | June 14, 199x | X-ray No.: | 43200 |
| Physician: | Harold B. Cooper, M.D. | Age: | 19 |
| Examination: | PA Chest, Abdomen | Hospital No.: | 90-32-11 |
| | | Room No.: | 1308 |

Findings:

PA CHEST:    Upright PA view of the chest shows the lung fields are clear, without evidence of an active process. Heart size is normal.

There is no evidence of a pneumoperitoneum.

IMPRESSION:    Negative chest.

ABDOMEN:    Flat and upright views of the abdomen show a normal gas pattern withou evidence of obstruction or ileus. There are no calcifications or abnormal masses noted.

IMPRESSION:    Negative study.

Radiologist  _____
Marian B. Skinner, M.D.

mtf
D:  6-14-9x
T:  6-14-9x

## 19—19 RADIOTHERAPY REPORTS

**_DO_**  type on a printed form or on plain paper the name of the patient, the date, and the name of the physician requesting the consultation. If a hospital case, type in the room number and hospital number.

**_DO_**  type single-spaced with main headings, whether dictated or not.

X-ray interpretation
Consultation
Therapy (specific preparation of the patient, identity, date, and amount of radiopharmaceutical medications used).

Figure 19–8 shows an example of a radiation therapy consultation report.

## 19—20 REFERENCE INITIALS

**_DO_**  use a double space below the typed signature line and type flush with the left margin.

**_DO_**  type the dictator's, the signer's, and the typist's initials when the dictator differs from the person who signs the medical report. Refer to Rule 19–1 when two medical examiners are involved in an autopsy protocol.

mjp/lrc/wpd  *or*  mjp:lrc:wpd
(Here, *mjp* stands for the dictator, *lrc* stands for the signer, and *wpd* stands for the typist.)

**Figure 19–8.** Radiotherapy Report generated from a hospital, typed in report form and in run-on format.

---

College Hospital
4567 Broad Avenue
Woodland Hills, XY 12345

RADIATION THERAPY CONSULTATION

Name: Theodore V. Valdez          Requested by: John L. Morris, M.D.

MR# 380780          Rm # 499          Date: 6/15/9x

HISTORY OF PRESENT MEDICAL ILLNESS: This is a 72-year-old who underwent decompressive laminectomy and Harrington rod placement in 1986 for angiosarcoma. Postoperative radiation therapy at Midway Hospital (Camarillo): 4025 cGy[1] in 23 fractions (175 cGy), 4 treatments per week, 2 to 1 PA to AP portals measuring 13 × 9 cm at 100 SSD on 8 Mv Linac, 5 HVL cord block at 3000 cGy. Dr. Davis estimates coverage T2 to T8. Myelogram and CT scan negative two years ago. However, developed cough and hemoptysis in past month. Chest x-ray and CT: right perihilar mass extending into mediastinum with multiple central and one anterior mediastinal mass with postobstructive infiltrate, bilateral pleural effusion. Bronchoscopy: 75% narrowing right upper lobe orifice to subsegments, 50% narrowing right lower lobe orifice. Bleeding at right upper lobe orifice. Draining right pleural effusion and sclerodesis with negative cytology. However, preliminary tissue diagnosis from right paratracheal area and mediastinoscopy: probable angiosarcoma.

PAST MEDICAL HISTORY: Hypertension.

SOCIAL HISTORY: 50 years tobacco habit.

PHYSICAL EXAMINATION: General: Well-developed male in no acute distress. No palpable adenopathy. Lungs: Clear. Heart: Regular rate and rhythm. Abdomen: Unremarkable. Extremities: Without circulatory collapse and edema. Neurologic: Without focal deficit.

ASSESSMENT: Recurrent metastatic angiosarcoma with postobstructive pneumonitis and hemoptysis.

PLAN: 4000 cGy[1] to symptom producing mediastinal disease. Initial 1000 cGy at 200 cGy fractions then oblique off previously irradiated spinal cord and boost with 250 cGy fractions. No plans for chemotherapy.

(continued)

---

1. cGy means centigray, and the abbreviation can also be typed CGy.

Page 2
Theodore V. Valdez
MR # 380780
June 15, 199x

PLAN: (continued)

Discussed radiation therapy procedures, risks, and alternatives with patient, emphasizing possible long-term risks to spinal cord, lung, and
heart as well as increased potential for morbidity resulting from prior irradiation. He agrees with treatment as outlined.

Sincerely,



Barry T. Goldstein, M.D.
Radiology Medical Group, Inc.

mtf
D: 6-15-9X
T: 6-16-9x

**DON'T** use humorous or confusing combinations of reference
initials.

crc (rather than cbc or cc)
db (rather than dmb)
dg (rather than dog)

19—21   SIGNATURE LINE

*DO* type 4 to 6 lines between the end of the report and the
signature line.

*DO* type the dictator's name. It is optional to insert a line
for the signature.

## 19—22    SPACING OF HEADINGS

**_DO_**    use double spacing or a space and a half between the last line of one heading and the next heading. It is optional to use no space below the main topic. Headings not dictated should be inserted.

## 19—23    STATISTICAL DATA

**_DO_**    include the information and use the format preferred by your employer and/or hospital facility.

## 19—24    SUBHEADINGS

**_DO_**    type in all capitals or upper- and lower-case followed by a colon. It is optional to begin each subtopic on a separate line. Headings not dictated may be inserted, but this too is optional.

## 19—25    TITLES OR MAJOR HEADINGS

**_DO_**    begin titles or major headings centered or at the left margin, depending on the preference of your employer and/or hospital facility. Type in all capital letters. It is optional to underline the title. Titles might be _Autopsy Protocol, Consultation, Discharge Summary, Operative Report, Pathology Report, Radiology Report,_ and so forth.

# 20

# Memos,

# MINUTES,

# AND

# OTHER

# REPORTS

## 20—1    AGENDA

The agenda is prepared before a meeting and establishes the order of business of the meeting and the items to be discussed or the plan of activities. It may be mailed to the membership well before the meeting or distributed as the meeting begins. The secretary will be able to use a copy to assist in taking notes and preparing the minutes.

The format of the agenda should be functional and easy to read. These goals are achieved by using layout techniques such as centered headings, columnar lists for agenda items and white space between items.The agenda should be typed, double-spaced and kept to one page if possible. Roman numerals are often used to number the items. The following information may be included in a formal agenda:

255

1. The name, date and time of the meeting (centered on the page).
2. The location of the meeting.
3. Call to order.
4. Roll call and/or introduction of members and/or board of directors.
5. Introduction of guests and/or new members.
6. Reading and approval of the minutes of the previous meeting.
7. Officers' reports. This is the main topic, and the individual reports are listed as subtopics.
8. Committee reports. This is the main topic, and the individual committee reports are listed as subtopics.
9. Old business. Unfinished business from the previous meeting is included. *Old Business* is the main topic, and the individual topics constituting old business are listed as subtopics.
10. New business. This is the main heading, and the individual topics (when known) constituting new business are listed as subtopics. Additional space is allowed at this point so that new topics may be added shortly before the meeting (at the president's discretion) or during the meeting itself.
11. Announcements. Often includes when and where the next meeting will be held.
12. Adjournment.

Figure 20–1 provides a sample formal agenda, and Figure 20–2 provides a sample informal agenda.

## 20—2    MEMORANDUMS

**Introduction:**    The purpose of the memorandum is to send information to one or more people within the office, company, division, department, or hospital, quickly and economically, in any situation in which written communication is appropriate. Memos are less formal than letters, and they also differ from letters in that they deal with routine information communicated between members of the same organization. Consequently, less background information is necessary.

AGENDA

TEAM MEDICAL MANAGEMENT PROGRAM

May 9, 199X

I. Call to Order

II. Roll Call and introduction of guests

James Morgan, M.D., representative from
Bayville Hospital

III. Approval of Minutes of April 14, 199X

IV. Officers' Reports

Treasurer's report

V. Committees

1. Bylaws Committee
2. Membership Committee
3. Nominating Committee
4. Credentials Committee

VI. Old Business
1. Attendance
2. Proposed changes in meeting time or day
3. Special project funding

VII. New Business
1. Health Fair (Dr. Dunn)
2. Evaluation of treadmill (Dr. Patton)
3. Discussion of 199X vacation schedules (Dr. Majur)

VIII. Announcements

Position open at Desert View Community. See Ron Miller.

Next meeting: Wednesday, June 18, 3 p.m., Board Room
(subject to approval today)

IX. Adjournment

**Figure 20–1.** Sample of a formal agenda.

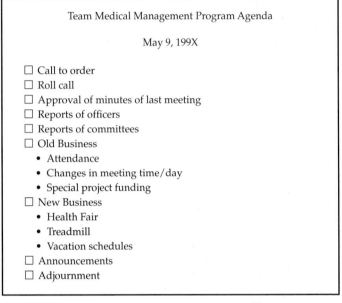

Figure 20–2. Sample of an informal agenda. Boxes (☐) introduce main headings, and bullets (•) introduce subheadings.

## Format

**Preprinted Forms:** Care must be taken to match the bottom of each line of typing with the bottom of each line of printing. One may use a variable line spacer to achieve this alignment. The distance between each printed line may determine the spacing of the rest of the memo. Memos are generally single-spaced.

**Typed Format:** Use plain, inexpensive paper and type out the appropriate headings. Set tab stops two or three spaces after the longest guide word in each column so that the information is vertically aligned. This format is preferred when additional space is required for the list of the persons receiving the memo.

**DATE:**     type out in full the date of origination. Sometimes this is typed in the position of the date line of a letter typed in modified block format, just to the right of the midline of the paper rather than lined up with the other headings as you see here.

**TO:**        a list of all the names of the persons or departments for routing the memo. A professional title may be used with the name, followed by the department, branch, and floor if deemed necessary.

**FROM:**    author, writer, dictator of the document.

**SUBJECT:**  the specific and accurate topic of the memo.

## Headings

The headings may be vertical or horizontal depending on the company's or typist's preference.

*VERTICAL:*
          DATE:
          TO:
          FROM:
          SUBJECT:

*HORIZONTAL:*
          TO:              DATE:
          FROM:            SUBJECT:

## Vertical Set-up

The headings are typed flush with the left margin, in full caps followed by a colon. Begin typing the headings two inches from the top of the paper, and double-space between headings. Set a tab 12 spaces in from the left margin, and tab over to fill in the headings.

Triple space and then begin the body of the memo.

The body of the memo is single spaced, with a double space between paragraphs. Use full-block format.

Figure 20–3 provides a sample of the vertical style memo.

## Horizontal Set-up

Type the first two headings flush with the left margin, double-space between the headings. Tab over eight spaces from the left margin to fill in the name of the recipient(s) of the memo, and repeat to fill in the name of the author. Type DATE and SUBJECT just to the right of the center of the page. From the first letter of DATE tab over 12 spaces to begin typing the date, and repeat to fill in the name of the subject. You can see that this format is not as easy to do as the more popular vertical style and could be inappropriate if the subject line is lengthy. Triple-space down to the body of the memo and complete as described for the vertical style.

Figure 20–4 provides a sample of a horizontal style memo.

MEMORANDUM

DATE:          January 14, 199X

TO:            Joan M. Abbott
               Shirley N. Andrews
               Martin P. Dorley

FROM:          Michael Jones, M.D.

SUBJECT:       Office Procedure Manual

It has come to my attention that when someone is sick or leaves on vacation, it is difficult to know how to complete certain tasks in the office. Therefore, I would like for each of you to work on a procedure manual for your specific job in this office, outlining from A–Z exactly what tasks you perform and how to carry them out.

The following activities should be listed:

1. Daily duties.
2. Weekly duties.
3. Monthly duties.
4. Quarterly duties.
5. Yearly duties.
6. Job attitudes.
7. Skills required for the job.
8. Clothing requirements.

Please have this ready by April 1. Thank you.

sna

**Figure 20–3.** A sample of the vertical style memo.

MEMORANDUM

TO: Joan M. Abbott          DATE:          January 14, 19XX
Shirley N. Andrews
Martin P. Dorley

FROM: Michael Jones, M.D.          SUBJECT: Office Procedure
                                             Manual

It has come to my attention that when someone is sick or leaves on vacation, it is difficult to know how to complete certain tasks in the office. Therefore, I would like each of you to work on a procedure manual for your specific job in this office, outlining from A–Z exactly what tasks you perform and how to carry them out.

The following activities should be listed:

1. Daily duties.
2. Weekly duties.
3. Monthly duties.
4. Quarterly duties.
5. Yearly duties.
6. Job attitudes.
7. Skills required for the job.
8. Clothing requirements.

Please have this ready by April 1. Thank you.

sna

**Figure 20–4.** A sample of the horizontal style memo.

## Lists

The following rules apply to listing in memos, reports, minutes, or policies.

1. Lists may be introduced with serial numbers or letters of the alphabet followed by a period or parentheses. Bullets (•) are also appropriate substitutes for numbers or letters.
2. Lists are typed in block format under the beginning of each line, and typing is not brought back under the number, letter, or bullet.
3. Lists do not need to be complete sentences but should be terminated with periods.
4. Lists should have parallel construction and be grammatically consistent, e.g., each line beginning with a verb: *type, list, spell, space*; or each line beginning with a noun or pronoun: *who, what, when, where*; or each line being a complete sentence.

## Closing Elements

The memo is completed with the typist's initials a double space after the last line of the body of the memo. It is not necessary to type the author's initials, but one should do so if it is the custom in the organization. A typed signature line is not used, nor does the author/dictator sign the memo.* Even though the memo is not signed by the author, it should always be submitted to him or her for approval before being distributed. Some writers will initial their memo after their name on the FROM line. Reference initials, enclosures, and copy notations should be handled exactly as they are in a letter: reference initials are typed two blank lines below the closing, then the enclosure line, followed by the copy notation, followed by the postscript, in that order, one or two blank lines below one another.

* There is a trend toward omitting the FROM line in favor of a typed signature at the close of the memo. If you choose this less formal approach, the author may initial or sign the memo here.

## Continuations

If the memo continues to an additional page or pages, begin typing one inch down from the top of the page and type in your headings: name of the addressee, date, and page number. Triple-space and continue with the body of the memo.

## 20—3  MINUTES

In order to assist the person recording minutes, one might set up a prepared standardized form that can be used to fill in information as the meeting is conducted. This also serves as a reminder to the note taker to be certain that important data are recorded. These are fairly easy to format on either typewriters or word processors and reflect the items found in the agenda. Figure 20–5 provides a sample prepared form.

Minutes are the formal or informal records of an organization's meeting and become the official documentation of what transpires during a meeting. They are usually taken by the recording secretary, although anyone attending the meeting may take minutes. It is helpful for the secretary to have the minutes of the previous meeting, a list of the membership, and the agenda for the meeting. The detail with which the notes are taken (or tape recorded) will be determined by the organization itself and the business conducted. It follows then that the content of the minutes will reflect the necessary detail. Whether the recorder merely summarizes the discussions or cites the speakers by name will be determined by the policy of the organization itself.

**Title.**   The heading is usually centered on the page and typed in full capital letters. It may be underlined as well.

**Date, Time, and Place.**   Date, time, and place of the meeting may be part of the heading or part of the report itself. The presiding officer is identified with the *call to order* or adjournment notation.

**Names of the Members.**   Names of the members present as well as members absent are listed in the minutes. If roll is taken, that sheet may be attached to the minutes. The names are usually listed in alphabetic order. List the names and include appropriate titles and other identifying information of any ex officio members or guests in attendance.

**Form for Recording Minutes**

Name of organization _____

Date _____ Time _____ Place _____

Present _____

_____

_____

Absent _____

Guests _____

Minutes _____

Officers' reports _____

Committee reports _____

_____

_____

Old Business _____

_____

_____

New Business _____

_____

_____

Announcements _____

Next Meeting _____

**Figure 20–5.** Sample form for recording minutes.

**Format.** The format should be consistent from meeting to meeting and secretary to secretary. The events should be reported in the order in which they occurred during the meeting. Outline format should be followed using the full block, modified block, or indented styles. The titles of the sections follow those of the agenda used at the meeting itself. Roman numerals are often used to introduce the titles of each section. Generally, headings (with or without numbers) should be typed flush with the left margin. Single-space the material under the headings and double space between headings. The headings are typed either in full capitals and underlined or with just the initial letter of the main words capitalized and the entire heading underlined.

The following items should be included: approval of minutes of the previous meeting; records of all officer and committee reports; records of all motions, seconds, etc.; action on any unfinished business; record of new business; announcements, including the date, time, and place of the next meeting; and the time of adjournment.

If the minutes continue to more than one page, the word *continued* may be typed at the bottom of the completed page. The subsequent page or pages begin an inch from the top of the page with the title of the minutes, the page number, and any other important data.

**Listing.** See *Lists* under Rule 20–2, *Memorandums*, for rules on listing.

**Closing.** The salutation *Respectfully submitted* followed by a triple space and the originator's name closes the minutes. The typist identifies the preparation of the document with a two- or three-letter identification, i.e., initials, a double space at the end, flush with the left margin.

**Distribution.** The minutes should be typed as soon as possible after the meeting and a copy distributed to all members (those present at the meeting and those absent) unless it is the custom to read the minutes at the following meeting. Some committees or organizations have a special distribution list that will include anyone who needs to be aware of the proceedings.

Figures 20–6 and 20–7 provide samples of informal minutes.

**Figure 20–6.** Sample of minutes.

---

Desert View Hospital                                    Mirage, Arizona

SAFETY COMMITTEE

MINUTES

DATE:

A meeting of the Safety Committee was called to order at 2:05 p.m. on August 22, 199X, in the Board Room.

MEMBERS PRESENT:

Bob Duncan, Rita Hardin, Jack Herzog, Pam Hollingsworth, Bobbie Lee, Dave Leithoff, Terri Peters, Carolyn Rath, Roland Wolf, and Joan Yubetta.

MEMBERS ABSENT:

Absent and excused were Carolyn Germano, Mary Harreld, and Peter Hulbert.

GUESTS:

Marijane Moss, RN, Pediatrics Unit.

MINUTES:

The minutes of the previous meeting were read. Bobbie Lee's name was added to the list of members present for the July 26 Safety Committee Meeting. The minutes were then approved as corrected.

ELECTRICAL SAFETY PROGRAM:

Joan Yubetta suggested that an electrical safety program be started. Rita Hardin reported that electrical cords are not being taped down.

(continued)

---

*Illustration continued on next page*

**Figure 20–6.** *continued*

---

Safety Committee Minutes
August 22, 199X
Page 2

FIRE DRILLS:

Dave Leithoff reported that there had been no fire drill in a month and suggested that there should be one by the end of September.

FIRST AID:

Terri Peters reported a total of 36 injuries for the month of August. Back injuries were down to five for August. There were seven falls, three cuts, and one foreign body.

It was suggested by Bob Duncan and Terri Peters that a form be designed for reporting scratches, puncture wounds, etc.

ADJOURNMENT:

There being no further business, the meeting was adjourned at 4:15 p.m. by Bob Duncan, Chairperson.

Respectfully submitted,

_____

Dave Leithoff, Recording Secretary

lro

---

**Figure 20–7.** Sample of minutes.

---

Desert View Hospital
Safety Committee

MINUTES

A meeting of the Safety Committee was called to order at 2:05 p.m. on August 22, 199X, in the Board Room.

I.   ROLL CALL

MEMBERS PRESENT:

> Bob Duncan, Rita Hardin, Jack Herzog, Pam Hollingsworth, Bobbie Lee, Dave Leithoff, Terri Peters, Carolyn Rath, Roland Wolf, and Joan Yubetta.

MEMBERS ABSENT:

> Absent and excused were Carolyn Germano, Mary Harreld, and Peter Hulbert.

GUESTS:

> Marijane Moss, RN, Pediatrics Unit.

II.  MINUTES:

> The minutes of the previous meeting were read. Bobbie Lee's name was added to the list of members present for the July 26 Safety Committee Meeting. The minutes were then approved as corrected.

III. REPORTS:

ELECTRICAL SAFETY PROGRAM:

> Joan Yubetta suggested that an electrical safety program be started. Rita Hardin reported that electrical cords are not being taped down.

---

*Illustration continued on next page*

**Figure 20–7.** *continued*

FIRE DRILLS:

Dave Leithoff reported that there had been no fire drill in a month and suggested that there should be one by the end of September.

FIRST AID:

Terri Peters reported a total of 36 injuries for the month of August. Back injuries were down to five for August. There were seven falls, three cuts, and one foreign body.

It was suggested by Bob Duncan and Terri Peters that a form be designed for reporting scratches, puncture wounds, etc.

IV.  ADJOURNMENT:

There being no further business, the meeting was adjourned at 4:15 p.m. by Bob Duncan, Chairperson.

Respectfully submitted,

_____

Dave Leithoff, Recording Secretary

lro

## 20—4    OUTLINES

Outlines are traditionally set up as shown in Figure 20–8. Remember that you must have at least two divisions or subdivisions in each set or a set cannot be made. Roman numerals, Arabic numerals, and letters of the alphabet are combined to identify different heading levels. A period and a double space follow each number or letter of the alphabet except at the levels where the parentheses are used, at which point you double-space after the closing parenthesis. The outlines are indented so that successive levels are obvious. One must leave space to backspace from the main topics in order to accommodate the width of the roman numerals. It is helpful to use the decimal tab set to align these numerals properly.

## 20—5    REPORTS AND POLICIES

See also Chapter 14, *History and Physical Format*, and Chapter 19, *Medical Reports*.

Reports and policies, just like minutes, have individual headings for the topics and titles. Unlike minutes, these will vary just as the nature of the report will vary. The originator of a report may or may not formulate the title for the transcriptionist, so he/she should be able to extract the title from the paragraph itself by pulling out the main idea and composing a brief heading for that section. The hospital or institution will usually have a special format, often special paper, for typing these documents.

**Headings.** Headings should be consistent throughout the report and follow simple guidelines:

1. Title: full caps spaced.
2. Main topics: full caps underlined.
3. Subtopics: full caps not underlined.
4. Minor topics: upper- and lower-case underlined.

**Listing.** See *Lists* under Rule 20–2, *Memorandums*, for rules on listing.

TITLE CENTERED AND TYPED IN FULL CAPS

I. Main Topic (first item) (Capitalize the first letter of each important word.)

    A. Secondary heading (Capitalize the first letter and any
    B. . . .                     proper nouns here and at all
    C. . . .                     other levels.)
    D. . . .

        1. Third level heading
        2. . .
        3. . .
        4. . .

           a. Fourth level heading
           b. . . .

              (1) Fifth level heading
              (2). . . .
              (3). . . .

                 (a) Sixth level heading
                 (b). . . .

II. Main Topic (second item) (You will have to backspace once

    A. . . .                     to allow for the roman numeral —
    B. . . .                     for balance.)
    C. . . .

      1. . . .
      2. . . .

    D. . . .

      1. . . .
      2. . . .
      3. . . .

III. Main Topic (third item) (You will have to backspace twice on this line for balance.)

The major headings and subdivisions may be a single word or phrase; long phrases or clauses; complete sentences; or any combination of sentences, phrases, and single words.

Between-line spacing is as follows:
    After title: triple-space.
    Main topic: double-space before and after each one.
    Subdivision items: single-space.
    Very brief outline: double-space all.

Indenting is as follows:
    Roman numerals: align to the left margin
    Division under each topic: set tab stops for four-space indent
    Second line: begin the second line of an item directly under
        the first letter of that line

**Figure 20–8.** Outline mechanics.

**Multipage Reports.** If a policy or report continues to more than one page, the word *continued* may be typed at the bottom of the completed page. The subsequent page or pages begin an inch from the top of the page with the title of the document, the page number, and any other important data (the policy number, for instance).

**Closing Format.** Figures 20–9 and 20–10 illustrate a simple report or policy closing format.

| | |
|---|---|
| Approved _____<br>        (Name) | Policy Number _____ |
| Effective date: | Revised: |
| Reviewed: | Revised: |

**Figure 20–9.** Sample closing policy format.

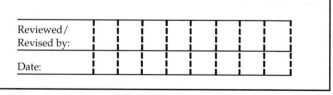

**ALVARADO HOSPITAL MEDICAL CENTER**

DEPARTMENT OF NURSING SERVICES

Date:

Approved:

Page: 1 of

PROCEDURE:

| Reviewed/ Revised by: | | | | | | | | | |
| --- | --- | --- | --- | --- | --- | --- | --- | --- | --- |
| Date: | | | | | | | | | |

**Figure 20–10.**  Sample format for a hospital procedure or policy.

# 21

# Metric

## SYSTEM

International System of
Units (SI) and Other
Forms of Measurement

## 21—1    ENGLISH MEASUREMENT

The use of abbreviations with the English form of measurement
is optional. When you do abbreviate, follow these rules.

**_DO_**         use the ' symbol for *foot* and " symbol for *inches* if
             desired in technical typing and tables.

**DON'T**    make these abbreviations plural or use punctuation
             marks with them (unless a word itself is formed
             when unpunctuated).

**DON'T** use an abbreviation unless it is expressed with a number.

*DO* use the following abbreviations for these common English measurements:

| | |
|---|---|
| ft **or** ' | foot |
| in. **or** " | inch (punctuate this one) |
| yd | yard |
| pt | pint |
| qt | quart |
| oz | ounce |
| fl oz | fluid ounce |
| gal | gallon |
| lb | pound |
| grain | grain (do not abbreviate) |
| dram | dram (do not abbreviate) |
| tsp **or** T | teaspoon |
| tbsp | tablespoon |
| c | cup |
| F | Fahrenheit |

The patient is 57 in. tall.
The patient is 57 inches tall.
The patient is 57" tall.

The baby's birth weight was 7 lb 3 oz.
The baby's birth weight was 7 pounds 3 ounces.

Further illustration of the use of measurements will be found in Chapter 22, *Numbers.*

## SI MEASUREMENT

The American spelling for all SI (metric) units will be used throughout, since that is preferred in the United States, that is, *meter* rather than the French *metre, liter* rather than *litre.*

## 21—2  SI BASE UNITS

| Unit | Symbol | Measures | Replaces |
|------|--------|----------|----------|
| meter | m | length, thickness | inch, foot, yard, mile |
| kilogram | kg | mass (weight) | ounce, pound |
| liter | L | volume | cup, pint, quart, gallon |
| Celsius | C | temperature | Fahrenheit |

There are other base units in the metric (SI) system, but they are not used frequently in daily life so are not dealt with in this chapter.

## 21—3  GENERAL RULES FOR SI MEASUREMENT

*DO*  write all abbreviations in small letters except for *C* for Celsius and *L* for liter.

**DON'T**  use abbreviations unless used with a number.

There was only about a mm difference. (incorrect)
There was only about a millimeter difference. (correct)

**DON'T**  combine a name with a symbol. When two or more names or symbols are used together, they should be spelled out in full or used in abbreviated form.

The temperature is 36°C. (correct)
The temperature is 36 degrees Celsius. (correct)
The temperature is 36 degrees C. (incorrect)
The temperature is 36°Celsius. (incorrect)
The temperature is 36° C. (incorrect spacing)

**DON'T**  use commas in large numbers.

53,471 (incorrect)
53 470 (correct)

**_DO_**  use a zero in front of the decimal point if the number is less than 1.

.57 (incorrect)
0.57 (correct)

.1 (incorrect)
0.1 (correct)

**DON'T**  use common fractions with the metric system.

1/4 cm (incorrect)
0.25 cm (correct)

1 3/4 L (incorrect)
1.75 L (correct)
1750 ml (correct)

**_DO_**  leave a space between the number and the symbol.

25mg (incorrect)
25 mg (correct)

0.4L (incorrect)
0.4 L (correct)

**_EXCEPTION._**  *Degrees Celsius is properly written with no spaces between numbers or abbreviations.*

37°C is normal body temperature.

*or*

37 degrees Celsius is normal body temperature.

**DON'T**   make symbols plural, no matter how many.

> 35 meters:
> 35 ms (incorrect)
> 35 m (correct)

**DON'T**   follow the abbreviations with a period.

> 1000 ml. (incorrect)
> 1000 ml (correct)

> 36°C. (incorrect)
> 36°C (correct)

**_DO_**   use a hyphen to link a number and a unit when they are used as a modifier.

> There is a 10-degree difference now.
> We noticed a 2.5-kg weight gain.
> He gained 2.5 kg.

## 21—4   SI MEASURING LENGTH, DISTANCE, THICKNESS — METER

**_DO_**   use meter for measuring length, distance, or thickness. Large distances are measured in kilometers (km), short lengths or distances are measured in meters (m), small thicknesses are measured in centimeters (cm), and very small thicknesses are measured in millimeters (mm).

**_DO_**   use the abbreviation **m** for meter, **km** for kilometer (1000 times a meter), **cm** for centimeter (1/100 meter) and **mm** for millimeter (1/1000 meter).

# 21  METRIC SYSTEM

## 21—5 SI MEASURING MASS (WEIGHT) — KILOGRAM

**_DO_** use the kilogram for measuring mass. A large mass is measured in kilograms (kg), a small mass is measured in grams (g), and a very small mass is measured in milligrams (mg).

**_DO_** use the abbreviation **kg** for kilogram (1000 times a gram), **g** for gram, and **mg** for milligram (1/1000 gram).

## 21—6 SI MEASURING TEMPERATURE — CELSIUS

**_DO_** use degrees Celsius (°C) for measuring temperature. Sometimes the term _centigrade_ is used instead of Celsius. They are equal to the same unit, and Celsius is preferred.

**_DO_** use the abbreviation °**C** or write out **degrees Celsius** to express temperature.

## 21—7 SI MEASURING VOLUME — LITER

**_DO_** use the liter for measuring volume. Large volumes are measured in liters (L) and small volumes in milliliters (ml or mL).

**_DO_** use the abbreviation L for liter (the lower-case letter looks too much like the number one), and the abbreviations ml or mL for milliliter (l/1000 liter).

**DON'T**   use cc (cubic centimeter or cm$^3$) as a substitute for ml, even though the volumes are the same. (The abbreviation cc is an incorrectly derived unit that has been substituted for ml.)

## 21—8   SI PREFIXES COMMONLY USED

|  | Prefix | Symbol | Relation | Example |
|---|---|---|---|---|
| More Than | kilo- | k | 1000 units | 1 kilogram, 1000 gm |
| One of a Unit | hecto- | h | 100 units | 1 hectometer, 100 m |
| Less Than | deci- | d | 1/10th unit | 1 deciliter, 0.1 liter |
| One of a | centi- | c | 1/100th unit | 1 centimeter, 0.01 m |
| Unit | milli- | m | 1/1000th unit | 1 milliliter, 0.001 L |

There is more than one way of expressing a metric measurement. Thus 1.5 (m) meters is also expressed as 150 (cm) centimeters or 1500 (mm) millimeters. The least complex expression is usually chosen; however, tradition may also dictate which is chosen. (Of course the transcriptionist transcribes exactly what is dictated, not making a "choice.")

## 21—9   MISCELLANEOUS DERIVED SI UNITS

**_DO_**   use these abbreviations for these derived units.

| | | |
|---|---|---|
| Hz | hertz | frequency |
| J | joule | energy |
| W | watt | power |
| V | volt | electric potential |

A metric conversion table (Table 21–1) is provided for your reference.

# 21 Metric System

## Table 21–1 Metric Conversions

| | When You Know | You Can Find | Symbols | If You Multiply by |
|---|---|---|---|---|
| **Length** | inches | millimeters | ml | 25 |
| | feet | centimeters | cm | 30 |
| | yards | meters | m | 0.9 |
| | miles | kilometers | km | 1.6 |
| | millimeters | inches | in | 0.04 |
| | centimeters | inches | in | 0.4 |
| | meters | yards | yd | 1.1 |
| | kilometers | miles | mi | 0.6 |
| **Area** | square inches | square centimeters | $cm^2$ | 6.5 |
| | square feet | square meters | $m^2$ | 0.09 |
| | square yards | square meters | $m^2$ | 0.8 |
| | square miles | square kilometers | $km^2$ | 2.6 |
| | acres | square hectometers (hectares) | ha | 0.4 |
| | square centimeters | square inches | $in^2$ | 0.16 |
| | square meters | square yards | $yd^2$ | 1.2 |
| | square kilometers | square miles | $mi^2$ | 0.4 |
| | square hectometers (hectares) | acres | | 2.5 |
| **Mass** | ounces | grams | g | 28 |
| | pounds | kilograms | kg | 0.45 |
| | short tons (metric tons) | megagrams | | 0.9 |
| | grams | ounces | oz | 0.035 |
| | kilograms | pounds | lb | 2.2 |
| | megagrams | short tons (metric tons) | | 1.1 |
| **Liquid Volume** | ounces | milliliters | ml | 30 |
| | pints | liters | l | 0.47 |
| | quarts | liters | l | 0.95 |
| | gallons | liters | l | 3.8 |
| | milliliters | ounces | oz | 0.034 |
| | liters | pints | pt | 2.1 |
| | liters | quarts | qt | 1.06 |
| | liters | gallons | gal | 0.26 |
| | teaspoons | milliliters | ml | 5 |
| | tablespoons | milliliters | ml | 15 |
| | fluid ounces | milliliters | ml | 30 |
| | cups | liters | l | 0.24 |
| **Temperature** | degrees Fahrenheit | degrees Celsius | °C | 5/9 (after subtracting 32) |
| | degrees Celsius | degrees Fahrenheit | °F | 9/5 (then add 32) |

# 22

# Numbers

# 22 NUMBERS

## INTRODUCTION

We have the terms *numeral, Arabic numerals, Roman numeral, numeric term, cardinal number, ordinal number,* and *figure.* Each one describes a different way that numbers themselves are expressed or written. Numbers can be spelled out, written as figures, or written in a combination of a figure and a part of a word (e.g., 3rd).

*Numeral* and *Arabic numeral* mean the *figures* and combination of the figures 0, 1, 2, 3, 4, 5, 6, 7, 8, 9.

*Numeric term* refers to written-out numbers.

*Roman numerals* refer to the use of certain letters of the alphabet, most frequently the capital letters and combination of the letters I, V, X.

*Cardinal numbers* refer to the quantity of objects in the same class. It may be a whole number, a fraction, or a combination, e.g., 3 days, $15, and so forth.

*Ordinal numbers* express position, sequence, or order of items in the same class. They can be spelled out or written as a figure plus a word part, e.g., first, 1st, third, eleventh, 14th, and so forth.

## 22—1    ABBREVIATIONS

See also Rule 22–26, *Symbols and Numbers.*

**_DO_**    use figures when numbers are directly used with symbols or abbreviations.

| | | | |
|---|---|---|---|
| 6 lb 7 oz | 1 q.i.d. | 99°F | 2% |
| 15 mmHg | $10 | #14 Foley | 5 ft 3 in. |
| pH 6.5 | | | |

**_DO_**    leave a space between the number and the abbreviation.

**DON'T**  leave a space between the number and the symbol.

> ***EXCEPTION.***  *Leave a space on either side of the ×  when used to mean* times *or* by.

I used a 3 × 5 card.

**DON'T**  combine a name with a symbol. When two or more names or symbols are used together, they should be spelled out in full or used in abbreviated form.

The temperature is 35°C. (correct)
The temperature is 35 degrees Celsius. (correct)
The temperature is 35 degrees C. (incorrect)
The temperature is 35° Celsius. (incorrect)
The temperature is 35 °C. (incorrect spacing)

***DO***  use figures with metric abbreviations.

| | | | |
|---|---|---|---|
| 1 mm | 10 cm | 0.5 mm | 7 ml |
| 20 kg | 37°C | 1 L | |

***DO***  use figures and symbols when writing plus or minus with a number.

pulses were 2+
presenting part was at a −2 station
use a +8.50 lens
a 2 to 3+ skin redundancy
1+ protein

## 22—2 ADDRESSES

**_DO_**  spell out the house number and post office box number **one** and the street numbers **one** through **ten**.

One East Wacker Drive
5060 Ninth Avenue
P.O. Box One

**_DO_**  use figures for all other house numbers, post office box numbers, and street and route names.

1335 11th Street
704 Worford Drive
P.O. Box 1178
Star Route 4

## 22—3 AGES

**_DO_**  use figures when expressing ages.

She had her first menses at age 12.
She is a 31-year-old police officer.
He is a 25-day-old infant.
He was 2 days 14 hours old.

**DON'T**  separate parts of the age with a comma.

He was 2 days, 14 hours old. (incorrect)

**DON'T**  use figures when expressing an indefinite age.

He was in his late fifties.
She started school at age four or five.

## 22—4   DATES

**_DO_**   use figures for the day of the month and the year; write out the month.

November 23, 1995 (conventional form)
23 November 1995 (military style)

**_DO_**   convert military style to conventional form in text formats.

He was born on 27 July. (incorrect)
He was born on 7/27. (incorrect)
He was born on July 27. (correct)

**_DO_**   use cardinal numbers (1, 2, 3, etc.) for expressing the date after the month and ordinal numbers (lst, 2nd, 3rd, etc./also 2d, 3d) for expressing the date before the month. The ordinal number is used with the date **only** before the name of the month.

She was first seen on the 2d of May. (correct)
She was first seen on the 2nd of May. (correct)
She was first seen on May 2. (correct)
She was first seen on May 2nd. (incorrect)
She was first seen on 2 May. (incorrect)

## 22—5   DECIMAL FRACTIONS

**_DO_**   use figures in writing numbers containing decimal fractions.

There was a 3.5 cm cut above the left eyebrow.

**_DO_**  express specific gravity with four digits and a decimal point. Place the decimal between the first and second digits.

The normal range for specific gravity in urine is 1.015–1.025.

**_DO_**  express temperature readings in decimal fractions when fractions are given.

98.6°F    35°

**_DO_**  place a zero before a decimal that does not contain a whole number. (Be very careful with the placement of the zero and decimal. Incorrect placement could result in a 10- or 100-fold error.)

The incision site was injected with 0.5% Xylocaine.

**_EXCEPTION._**  *He used a .22 caliber rifle.*

## 22—6    DIMENSIONS AND MEASUREMENTS

See also Chapter 21, *Metric System.*

**_DO_**  use figures and symbols when writing dimensions. Leave a space each side of the X. Use upper- or lower-case X, whichever looks best in the text.

two 4 × 4 sponges

The burn scar was 60 mm × 4 cm.

12 × 14 ft area

**_DO_**   add a zero after the decimal point and whole number for consistency in the set of numbers containing a decimal fraction.

$8.5 \times 5.0 \times 4.0$ (correct)
$8.5 \times 5 \times 4$ (incorrect)

## 22—7   DRUGS

**_DO_**   use figures in all expressions pertaining to drugs including strength, dosage, and directions.

He is to take Tofranil, 75 mg/day $\times$ 3 days to be increased to 100–150 mg/day if there is no response.

The directions for her Motrin were 400 mg q4h PRN pain.

One generally gives 6.2 mg/kg to 9.4 mg/kg for those children 9 years old or younger.

## 22—8   EKG LEADS

**_DO_**   use figures and abbreviations when writing electrocardiographic **chest** leads. (These leads are $V_1$ through $V_6$ and $aV_L$, $aV_R$, and $aV_F$.) They may be written properly with subscripts or on line when the subscript format is unavailable.

There is an ST elevation in leads V-2 and V-6.

*or*

There is an ST elevation in leads $V_2$ and $V_6$ .

# 22 NUMBERS

*NOTE.* *See Rule 22–21 for numbers used with* **limb** *leads.*

## 22—9  FRACTIONS

See also Rule 22–5, *Decimal Fractions.*

**DO**  spell out and hyphenate fractions standing alone.

He smoked a half-pack of cigarettes a day.
He smoked one-half pack of cigarettes a day.

There was a three-quarter inch difference between the two bones.

Paresis is noted in four-fifths of the left leg.

**DO**  use figures to write mixed numbers (whole numbers with a fraction).

1 1/2      7 5/8      6 3/4

## 22—10  INCLUSIVE (CONTINUED) NUMBERS

**DO**  use the hyphen to take the place of the word *to* or *through* to identify ranges.

Take 100 mg Tylenol, 1–2 h.s.

The L2–5 vertebrae were involved.

30–35 mEq

Rounds were made in Wards 1–4.

practicing there from 1980–1989

checked the records from the 400–450 series

She has a 50–50 chance.

Check $V_2$-$V_6$ again.

Cranial nerves II–XII were intact.

**DON'T** use a hyphen when one or both ends of the range contain a minus sign.

at a –2 to a –3 station

## 22—11 INDEFINITE EXPRESSIONS

*DO* write out numbers that are used for indefinite expressions.

I received thirty-odd applications.
He had diphtheria in his mid-forties.
Hundreds thronged to see my "celebrity" patient.
I had about a thousand reasons for doing that.
Several hundred doctors were expected to attend.
There was a five-fold increase in membership.

There were eighteen hundred physicians present at the symposium. (correct)

There were one thousand eight hundred present. (incorrect)

# 22 NUMBERS

## 22—12 LARGE NUMBERS

**_DO_**     express round numbers in the millions and billions in a combination of figures and words.

Do you know that Keane Insurance sold over $3 1/2 billion worth of medical insurance last year?

**_DO_**     use the exponential form of scientific notation for large scientific numbers above 1,000,000. Be sure to write the exponent in superscript.

$7^3$ (seven to the power of three)

**_DO_**     express large technical numbers in figures and punctuate appropriately (see Rule 6–16).

The culture grew 100,000 colonies of _E. coli_ per cubic centimeter.

The insurance reimbursement was $1240.

## 22—13 LISTS

**_DO_**     use serial figures for listing and enclose them in parentheses when enumerating in text material. Use serial figures followed by a period in a vertical list.

Plan on admittance: (1) Stat WBC, (2) Barium enema, (3) Urinalysis, (4) Routine chest x-ray.

Rule out:    1. Acute appendicitis.
             2. Ectopic pregnancy.
             3. Endometritis.
             4. Polycystic ovary.

22—14   MONEY

***DO***        use figures to express amounts of money.

She was offered a $27,000-a-year salary.

**DON'T**   use periods and zeros with whole dollar amounts unless two or more amounts are used in the same context in the sentence.

My consultation fee was $85.00, but the insurance reimbursement was just $45.37. (correct)

The initial consultation fee is $85. (correct)
The initial consultation fee is $85.00. (incorrect)

**DON'T**   use symbols for less than whole dollar amounts.

Please give her the 35 cents change. (correct)
Please give her the 35¢ change. (incorrect)
Please give her the $0.35 change. (incorrect)

***DO***        express round dollar amounts in the millions and billions in a combination of figures and words preceded by the dollar symbol.

Do you know that Keane Insurance sold over $3 billion worth of medical insurance last year?

***DO***        spell out indefinite amounts of money.

I think there was just a few dollars' difference.

He was offered several thousand dollars more to stay.

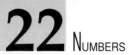

---

## 22—15    NAMES

---

**_DO_**    use roman numerals (I, II, etc.) or ordinals (2d, 3d, etc.) without punctuation after a person's surname, following the individual's preference.

Jon-Pierre Wolffstetter II

William Paul Denny 3d

---

## 22—16    NEIGHBORING AND RELATED NUMBERS

---

**_DO_**    use a figure for one number and spell out the other when two numbers are used together to modify the same noun. (Note also the use of the hyphen in the compound modifier.)

two l-liter solutions
six 3-bed wards
twenty 4 × 4 sponges

**_DO_**    use figures to write numbers less than ten when they are related to a large number on the same subject.

There are 3 beds available on the medical wing, 14 on the surgery wing, and 12 on the pediatric floor.

---

## 22—17    ORDINALS (First, Second, Third, etc.)

---

**_DO_**    spell out ordinals written as one or two words **except** when used as a date appearing **before** the month or in street numbers above ten.

The fourth, fifth, and sixth ribs were fractured.

He was a member of the Seventh-day Adventist church.

The patient was discharged to his home on the tenth postoperative day.

Give the patient an appointment for the 3d of August.

The office address is 1335 11th Street.

**DON'T**    space between the number and the *th, d,* or *st.*

**_DO_**    hyphenate compound ordinals.

the eighty-fifth congress

## 22—18   PLURALS

**_DO_**    form the plural of figures by adding *s.*

**DON'T**    use an apostrophe.

Be sure that your 2s don't look like z's.

**_DO_**    form the plural of written out numbers just as you form the plural of other words (see Chapter 25).

She moved here sometime in the forties.

He refused to do his serial 7s.

## 22—19    PUNCTUATION WITH NUMBERS

**_DO_**    use a colon between numbers to express ratios. The colon takes the place of the word *to*.

The solution was diluted 1:100.

**_DO_**    use a dash and parentheses with telephone numbers.

Call (800) 626–3126 between nine and five.

**_DO_**    use a colon between the hours and minutes indicating the time of day in figures.

The patient expired at 10:30 a.m.

**_DO_**    use a comma between a pair of numbers to facilitate reading the numbers and to avoid confusion.

In 1990, 461 cases were reviewed by the Tumor Board.

**_DO_**    use a comma to set off a year date that is used to explain a preceding date of the month.

He was born on March 3, 1933, in Reading, Pennsylvania.

**_DO_**    use commas to group numbers in units of three.

300,000 units    platelets 250,000    wbc 15,000
1,567,988

*EXCEPTION.* Numbers used with metric measurements, telephone numbers, social security numbers, insurance and other ID numbers, addresses, credit card numbers, and binary notation (a combination of 0's and 1's).

100100101    526-98-8543    JTY 7894A
24987 Sepulveda Drive

*DO*        use a hyphen to join numbers to words in a compound modifier.

6-kg weight        35-mm film
4-mm-thick layer    2-week convalescence

**DON'T**    use commas or hyphens with four-digit numbers, the metric system, street numbers, dates, ZIP codes, and some ID and technical numbers unless they are actually part of the number.

My bill to Medicare was $1250.

1 000 ml (correct
1,000 ml (incorrect)

**DON'T**    use commas to separate two units of the same dimension.

The infant was 3 days 4 hours old.

She was a Gravida 4 Para 2 white female.

The surgery was completed in 2 hours 40 minutes.

He was 6 ft 3 in. tall. (Note the period after *in.* in the previous example. This abbreviation is punctuated since it can be misread as the word *in* rather than the abbreviation for *inch*.)

**_DO_**    use a hyphen to separate letters and words from numbers to describe chemical elements except with subscript or superscript.

Uranium-235      I-131

**_DO_**    use hyphens and close-up punctuation in chemical formulas.

9-nitroanthra(l,9,4,10)bix(1)osathiazone-2,7-bix-dioxide

**_DO_**    hyphenate numbers 21–99 when they are written out.

Fifty-five medical transcriptionists attended the meeting last night.

**_DO_**    use a hyphen to take the place of the word _to_ to identify numerical ranges.

Take 1–2 at bedtime.

The L2–5 vertebrae were involved.

30–35 mEq      a 50–50 chance

**DON'T**   repeat the symbol used in a range.

99–102° temperature

**_DO_**    use parentheses to separate numbers used in text. (see Rule 22–13, _Lists_).

## 22—20   RATIOS

***DO***      use a colon between numbers to express ratios. The colon takes the place of the word *to*.

The solution was diluted 1:100.

We had a 2:1 mix.

We used 1:6000 Adrenalin.


## 22—21   ROMAN NUMERALS

**DON'T**   use a type font that is sans serif (e.g., Chicago) because the capital letter **I** needed for Roman numerals looks like the number one.

***DO***      use Roman numerals to describe the twelve cranial nerves, the EKG limb leads, and the EEG cranial leads.

Cranial nerves II–XII were intact.
Cranial nerves II to XII were intact.

Cranial lead I was not responding properly.

The EKG limb lead III was disconnected.

***DO***      use Roman numerals with typical non-counting or non-mathematical listings. By tradition in medicine these include the following:

| Type | type I hyperlipoproteinemia |
| Factor | missing factor VII (blood factor) |
| Stage | stage II carcinoma |
| | stage I coma |
| | lues II (secondary syphilis) |
| | Billroth I (first stage of surgery) |
| Phase | phase II clinical trials |
| Class | class II malignancy |
| | cardiac status: Class IV |
| Grade | grade II systolic murmur |
| Technique | Coffey technique III |

| pregnancy and delivery | gravida III para II abortion 0 |
| with the Greek alphabet | alpha II |
| generations in family pedigree | subject 4 in generation II |
| personal names | W. Peter Wood III |

*NOTE. Proper nouns that accompany the Roman numeral must be capitalized. Other nouns are not capitalized unless they are at the beginning of a sentence, part of a set, or the initial word in an outline.*

\*OB/GYN:  Gravida VI Para IV Abortion II
            Gravida 6 Para 4 Abortion 2

There is a well-differentiated (FIGO Grade I) adeno-carcinoma.

(Notice in these examples that the rest of the words in the sets are also capitalized for consistency.)

**_DO_**    use Roman numerals for major divisions in an outline (see Figures 20–7 and 20–8).

---

\*Some professionals prefer the use of the arabic numerals with gravida and para.

## 22—22    SPACING WITH SYMBOLS AND NUMBERS

**_DO_**    type the following symbols directly in front of or directly following the number they refer to, with no spacing.

+, =, %, #, $, °, @, &, –, /

**_DO_**    space on each side of the × that takes the place of the word *times* or the word *by*.

## 22—23    SPELLED-OUT/WRITTEN-OUT NUMERIC TERMS

**_DO_**    spell out numbers at the beginning of a sentence (or reword the sentence to avoid beginning with a number).

> **NOTE.** *When several related numbers are used in a sentence, be consistent; type all numbers in figures or write them all out. Normally, it is easier to type all of them in figures. However, if you must begin a sentence with a written-out number, you are not bound to write out the other large numbers in the sentence.*

Seventy-one percent responded to the questionnaire; 33% were positive, 21% were negative, and 17% gave a "no opinion" response.

**_DO_**    remember to spell out an abbreviation or symbol used with a number if the number has to be spelled out for some reason (see previous example).

**_DO_**    spell out numbers one through and including ten when they do not refer to technical items and do not appear in the same sentence with larger numbers.

She had pulmonary tuberculosis three years ago and spent seven months in a sanatorium.

We had seven admissions Saturday and three already this morning.

**_DO_** spell out numbers that are used for indefinite expressions.

I received thirty-odd applications.
He had diphtheria in his mid-forties.

**_DO_** spell out fractions standing alone.

He smoked a half-pack of cigarettes a day.
Paresis is noted in four-fifths of the left leg.

**_DO_** spell out one number and use a figure for the other when two numbers are used together to modify the same noun.

two 1-liter solutions
six 3-bed wards
130 one-day admissions

**_DO_** spell out the even time of day when written with or without *o'clock* and without a.m. or p.m.

The staff meeting is scheduled to begin at three.

He is due at nine this evening.

Give her an appointment for two o'clock.

**DO** spell out large round numbers that do **not** refer to technical quantities.

There were eighteen hundred physicians present at the symposium.

He was given six hundred thousand units of penicillin. (Incorrect. This is a technical number.)

He was given 600,000 units of penicillin. (correct)

## 22—24 SUBSCRIPT AND SUPERSCRIPT

**DO** use subscript or superscript as appropriate in writing the following values:

*Superscript*
scientific notation
(seven to the power of ten)                     $7^{10}$

place the mass number                           $^{238}U$
in the superior position
to the left of the symbol.

glucose 14 C                                    $^{14}C$

See Table 22–1 for a list of radioactive pharmaceuticals.

*Subscript*
chemical elements and compounds
(oxygen)                                        $O_2$
(carbon dioxide)                                $CO_2$
vitamin components                              $B_{12}$
vertebral column                                $L_{4-5}$
(fourth and fifth lumbar)
chest leads                                     $V_1$–$V_6$
heart sounds                                    $A_2 P_2$

## Table 22–1. Symbols for Chemical Elements and Radioactive Pharmaceuticals

| Symbol | Element | Symbol | Element | Symbol | Element |
|---|---|---|---|---|---|
| Ac | actinium | Gd | gadolinium | Pr | praeseodymium |
| Ag | silver | Ge | germanium | Pt | platinum |
| Al | aluminum | H | hydrogen | Pu | plutonium |
|  | (aluminium) | Ha | hahnium | Ra | radium |
| Am | americium | He | helium | $^{226}$Ra |  |
|  |  | Hf | hafnium |  |  |
| $^{241}$Am |  | Hg | mercury | Rb | rubidium |
| Ar | argon | $^{197}$Hg |  | Re | rhenium |
| As | arsenic | $^{203}$Hg |  | Rf | rutherfordium |
| At | astatine | Ho | holmium | Rh | rhodium |
| Au | gold | I | iodine | Rn | radon |
| $^{198}$Au |  | $^{123}$I |  | $^{222}$Rn |  |
| B | boron | $^{125}$I |  | Ru | ruthenium |
| Ba | barium | $^{131}$I |  | $^{106}$Ru |  |
| Be | beryllium | In | indium | S | sulfur |
| Bi | bismuth | $^{111}$In |  | $^{35}$S |  |
| Bk | berkelium | $^{113m}$In |  | Sb | antimony |
| Ir | iridium |  |  | Sc | scandium |
| Br | bromine | K | potassium | Se | selenium |
| C | carbon | $^{42}$K |  | $^{75}$Se |  |
| $^{14}$C |  | Kr | krypton | Si | silicon |
| Ca | calcium | $^{85}$Kr |  | Sm | samarium |
| $^{47}$Ca |  | La | lanthanum | Sn | tin |
| Cd | cadmium | Li | lithium | Sr | strontium |
| Ce | cerium | Lr | lawrencium | $^{85}$Sr |  |
| Cf | californium | Lu | lutetium | $^{87m}$Sr |  |
| Cl | chlorine | Md | mendelevium | $^{90}$Sr |  |
| Cm | curium | Mg | magnesium | Ta | tantalum |
| Co | cobalt | Mn | manganese | Tb | terbium |
| $^{57}$Co |  | Mo | molybdenum | Tc | technetium |
| $^{60}$Co |  | N | nitrogen | $^{99m}$Tc |  |
| Cr | chromium | Na | sodium | Te | tellurium |
| $^{51}$Cr |  | $^{24}$Na |  | Th | thorium |
| Cs | cesium | Nb | niobium | Ti | titanium |
| $^{137}$Cs |  | Nd | neodymium | Tl | thallium |
| Cu | copper | Ne | neon | $^{201}$Tl |  |
| $^{64}$Cu |  | Ni | nickel | Tm | thulium |
| Dy | dysprosium | No | nobelium | U | uranium |
| Er | erbium | Np | neptunium | V | vanadium |
| Es | einsteinium | O | oxygen | W | tungsten |
| Eu | europium | Os | osmium | Xe | xenon |
| F | fluorine | P | phosphorus | $^{133}$Xe |  |
| $^{18}$F |  | $^{32}$P |  | Y | yttrium |
| Fe | iron | Pa | protactinium | Yb | ytterbium |
| $^{59}$Fe |  | Pb | lead | $^{169}$Yb |  |
| Fm | fermium | $^{210}$Pb |  | Zn | zinc |
| Fr | francium | Pd | palladium | Zr | zirconium |
| Ga | gallium | Pm | promethium |  |  |
| $^{67}$Ga |  | Po | polonium |  |  |

*NOTE.* *All of these expressions can be typed on the same line if your typing equipment is not capable of printing small numbers above or below the line, with the* **exception of scientific notation**.

V-4   L4–5   B12   $CO_2$   $O_2$   U-238   14C   A-2  P-2

## 22—25   SUTURE MATERIALS

In the USP system, sutures range in size from the smallest (11-0), which are described with the appropriate number of zeros, to the largest (7), which are described as #1 through #7. In the Brown & Sharp (B & S) sizing of stainless steel sutures, the range is from the smallest (#40) through the largest (#20).

*DO*        use figures in writing suture materials.

*NOTE.* *When the dictator says "three oh" or "triple oh" in referring to suture materials, you may type 000 or 3-0. For reading ease, use only the number, hyphen and the zero when the number is larger than three, that is, from 4-0 through 11-0.*

The incision was closed with #6-0 fine silk sutures. (correct)
The incision was closed with #000000 fine silk sutures. (incorrect)
The incision was closed with #60 fine silk sutures. (incorrect)

She used 000 chromic catgut for suture material. (correct)
She used 3-0 chromic catgut for suture material. (correct)
She used #3-0 chromic catgut for suture material. (correct)
Please order a box of #l silk.

**_DO_**     be consistent throughout the report in describing the suture materials.

**DON'T**    confuse these markings with the Vicryl sutures or stainless steel sutures when a different gauge designation may be dictated.

The corneoscleral incision was closed with interrupted #70 Vicryl sutures.

A Bunnell 34-gauge pull-out wire was woven through the extensor tendon and tied over a button.

## 22—26    SYMBOLS AND NUMBERS

**_DO_**     use symbols in preference to the spelled-out word when they occur in immediate association with a number and are used to express technical terms.

| | |
|---|---|
| 8 × 3 | eight by three |
| 4–5 | four to five |
| #3-0 | number three oh |
| 2+ | two plus |
| Vision: 20/20 | vision is twenty-twenty |
| 6/day | six per day |
| diluted 1:10 | diluted one to ten |
| at −2 | at minus two |
| 60/40 | sixty over forty |
| Grade IV/V | grade four over five |
| nocturia × 2 | nocturia times two |
| 25 mg/hr | twenty-five milligrams per hour |
| limited by 45% | limited by forty-five percent |
| 35 mg% | thirty-five milligrams percent |
| 30°C | thirty degrees Celsius |
| 99°F | ninety-nine degrees Fahrenheit |
| BP: 100/80 | blood pressure is one hundred over eighty |

**DON'T**    use the degree symbol (°) in describing temperature if the word *degree* is not dictated or is not represented on your keyboard.

Temperature: 36 C. (correct)
Temperature: 36°C. (also correct)

**DON'T**    use the percent symbol (%) in nonscientific text.

Only a quarter of those invited were on time.

Only fifty percent arrived on time.

**DON'T**    use simple fractions with percent.

45 1/2 percent (incorrect)
45 1/2% (incorrect)
45.5% (correct)

22—27    TIME

*DO*    spell out the even time of the day when written with or without *o'clock* or without a.m. or p.m.

The staff meeting is scheduled to begin at *three*.
He is due at *nine* this evening.
Give her an appointment for *two* o'clock.
She was seen as an emergency at a *quarter past ten*.

*DO*    use figures to express the time of day with a.m. or p.m. and the time of day when both hours and minutes are expressed alone.

Office hours are from 10 a.m. to noon. Your appointment is for 11:30.

**DON'T**  use the colon and double zeros for even periods of time.

Office hours are from 10:00 a.m. to noon. (incorrect)
Office hours are from 10 a.m. to noon. (correct)

**DON'T**  Use the expression *o'clock* with *a.m.* or *p.m.*

She is expected at 3 o'clock p.m. (incorrect)
She is expected at three o'clock. (correct)

**DON'T**  use *a.m.* or *p.m.* with 12. You may use the figure 12 with the word *noon* or *midnight* or use the words alone without the figure 12.

We close the office at 12 noon.
My shift is over at midnight.

**_DO_**  use figures without a colon when writing the military time of day.

0315    (zero three fifteen — 3:15 a.m.)
1200    (twelve hundred hours — noon)
1400    (fourteen hundred hours — 2 p.m.)
1630    (sixteen thirty — 4:30 p.m.)

Your appointment is set for 16:30. (incorrect)
Your appointment is set for 1630. (correct)

**_DO_**  use the expression *o'clock* to refer to points on a circular surface, and use figures with *o'clock*.

The sclera was incised at about the 3 o'clock area.

The cyst was in the left breast, just below the nipple, between 4 and 5 o'clock.

Then 1:2 mL of 1% lidocaine was injected at the 4 o'clock and 8 o'clock positions.

**_DO_**     write out numbers to express _periods of time_ when the number is less than ten; when the number is over ten, use the figure.

She is to return in follow-up in three months' time.

The B-R Medical Supply invoice is marked "net 30 days."

## 22—28   UNRELATED NUMBERS

**_DO_**     follow the rules governing the use of each number when unrelated numbers appear in the same sentence.

He has _three_ offices and employs _21_ medical assistants, including _2_ transcriptionists.

## 22—29   VERTEBRAL COLUMN AND SPINAL NERVES

**_DO_**     use figures with capital letters to refer to the vertebral (spinal) column and spinal nerves as follows:

C           cervical 1–7
T (or D)  thoracic (or dorsal) 1–12
L           lumbar 1–5
S           sacral 1–5

He has a herniated disk at $C_{4-5}$.
He has a herniated disk at C4–5.

There was an injury to the spine
between $C_7$ and $T_1$.
There was an injury to the spine
between C7 and T1.

## 22—30   VISUAL ACUITY AND REFRACTIONS

***DO***   use figures and symbols to express visual acuity.

OD: $+3.25+0.75 \times 125 = 20/30-1$

vision was corrected to 20/200

***NOTE.*** *Use care in transcribing numbers that make sense. The above expression may have sounded like 22/100, which would not make sense.*

## 22—31   VITAL STATISTICS

***DO***   use figures in writing vital statistics such as age, weight, height, blood pressure, pulse, respiration, dosage, size, temperature, and so forth.

He is a 16-year-old, well-developed, well-nourished white male. Height: 72". Weight: 145 lb. Blood Pressure: 120/80. Pulse: 72. Respirations: 18.

The patient has 20/40 vision in his right eye and 20/100 in his left eye.

## 22—32   WORDS USED WITH NUMBERS

**_DO_**  use figures (Roman or cardinal) for numbers used in close association with words (see also Rule 22–21, *Roman Numerals* and Rule 4–12, *Numbers with Nouns*.)

#14 Foley catheter
No. 14 Foley catheter
Grass Ten Channel Serial #627-B
Medicare ID 527-40-7201A
Grade II systolic murmur

# 23

# PARENTHESES

## INTRODUCTION

Parentheses, commas, and dashes are all used to set off incidental or nonessential elements in text. Which you choose will be determined either by the dictator/writer of the material or by the closeness of the relationship between the material enclosed and the rest of the sentence. In general, commas are used to set apart closely related material slightly; parentheses are used when commas have already been used within the nonessential element or the material itself is neither grammatically nor logically essential to the main thought. The dash is a more forceful and abrupt division and draws attention to a statement; parentheses de-emphasize. Enclosed material can range from a single punctuation mark (!) to several sentences.

## 23—1    ENUMERATIONS

**_DO_**    use parentheses around figures or letters in enumerations indicating divisions.

(1)  Sterile field.
(2)  Suture materials.
(3)  4 × 4 sponges.

It is my impression that she has (1) progressive dysmenorrhea, (2) uterine leiomyoma, (3) weakness of the right inguinal ring.

I did not hire her for the medical assisting position because (a) she lacked enthusiasm, (b) her spoken grammar lacked polish, and (c) her typing speed was fairly low (45 wpm).

**NOTE.** *You may also use figures or letters followed by a period rather than enclosed in parentheses in enumerations except in narrative text material.*

1. Sterile field.
2. Suture materials.
3. 4 × 4 sponges.

## 23—2   EXPLANATIONS OR COMMENTS

**_DO_**   use parentheses to enclose material that is an explanation, definition, or comment.

Because of his condition (emphysema) and age (88), he is a poor risk for anesthesia at this time.

The patient felt that she had inhaled some sort of ornamental dust (gold, silver, bronze, etc.) while working in her flower shop.

The administrative medical assistant (receptionist, secretary, bookkeeper, insurance clerk, transcriptionist, file clerk) requires the same length of training as the clinical medical assistant.

He says he is a "doctor" (Ph.D.) and prefers to use that title.

**NOTE.** *A complete sentence enclosed within parentheses does not require a capital letter to open it nor a period to close it.*

Her temperature peaked at 106.5 degrees (we were relieved when this occurred) and the seizures subsided.

## 23—3   IDENTIFICATION

**DO** use parentheses to enclose an abbreviation after the first completely spelled-out use.

All newborns are routinely tested for phenylketonuria (PKU). As a result, the incidence of PKU as the cause of infant . . .

**DO** use parentheses to enclose the brand name of a drug after the proprietary name has been used in the text.

I would like to start him out on a nonsteroidal, anti-inflammatory agent such as ibuprofen (Motrin) or indomethacin (Indocin).

## 23—4   LEGAL DOCUMENTS

**DO** in preparation of medicolegal documents, place parentheses around numerals after a spelled-out figure.

The patient will not be permitted to return to his full usual and customary duties for a period of thirty-five (35) working days.

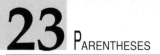

# 23 PARENTHESES

---

## 23—5　NONESSENTIAL ELEMENTS

---

**_DO_**　　use parentheses to set off words or phrases that are clearly nonessential to the sentence.

According to the pathology report (see enclosed), there is no evidence of active pulmonary tuberculosis at this time.

## 23—6　PUNCTUATION AND CAPITALIZATION

---

**_DO_**　　place punctuation marks outside of the material enclosed in parentheses unless it is needed at the end of a complete parenthetical sentence or for definition within the material itself. (See previous rules [23–1 through 23–5] for examples.)

**DON'T**　capitalize the beginning of a sentence when it occurs in parentheses within a sentence.

We are leaving for the workshop in Phoenix early tomorrow (**w**ho got me into this?), and we should be back by Friday evening.

We are leaving for the workshop in Phoenix early tomorrow, and we should be back by Friday evening. (**W**ho got me into this?)

Her temperature peaked at 106.5 degrees (we were relieved when this occurred), and the seizures subsided.

**_DO_** use dashes with parentheses when two or more overlapping parenthetical elements are used to interrupt the same sentence.

The debate concerning the approval of lay visitors to the Tumor Board Conference became heated — we had to recess several times (once for 40 minutes) — and we finally adjourned with no definitive policy established.

## 23—7   REFERENCES

**_DO_** use parentheses to enclose a reference notation.

A complete list of all the rules in this section is given on the first page of the chapter (see page 32).

Dr. Norman F. Billups is best known to medical transcriptionists as the author of the _American Drug Index_ (J.B. Lippincott).

D. Krathwohl, et al., _Taxonomy of Educational Objectives: Affective Domain_ (New York: David Mckay, 1964)

## 23—8   SCIENTIFIC USE

**_DO_** use parentheses to enclose certain mathematical elements, formulas, certain chemical and molecular components that must be grouped, immunoglobulin notations, and genetic notations concerning chromosomes.

Immunoglobulin notation: IgG(Pr)

Unknown sequences of amino acids in polypeptides: (Asp, His, Pro)

Biochemical conventions:
$(CH_3)_2CHCh_2Ch(NH_2)$   COOH

Symbolization for structurally altered chromosomes:
46,XX,t(4;13)(p21;q32)

## 23—9  SPACING

**DON'T** space after the left parenthesis or before the right parenthesis.

# Period and

# Decimal Point

## INTRODUCTION

The period is a mark of terminal punctuation. Some physicians from foreign countries dictate "full stop" when indicating the end of a sentence. Other dictators may say "period" or rely on voice inflection to indicate the end of a sentence.

## 24—1   ABBREVIATIONS

**_DO_**      use a period with some abbreviations as follows:

**Single capitalized words and single letter abbreviations with one space typed after the period:**

Mr.     Jr.     Dr.     Inc.     *E. coli*     *M. tuberculosis*
Joseph P. Myers

Mr. John A. Jeffreys Jr. was the guest speaker.

Academic degrees and religious orders with no spaces between the period and the next letter, one space after the period:

M.D.      Ph.D.      D.D.S.      B.V.E.
M.S.      O.S.A.     S.J.

Peter L. Montega, M.D., saw him in consultation early this morning.

Lower case Latin abbreviations with no spaces between the period and the next letter, one space after the period:

a.m.  p.m.  e.g.  t.i.d.  h.s.

**DON'T** use a period with the following lower-case abbreviations:

**Units of measurement:**
wpm  mph  ft  oz  sq in  ml  mL  cm

*EXCEPTION.*   *Don't use* in *for inch;* in. *is better.*

**Certification, registration, and licensure abbreviations:**

CMA-A  CMT  RN  RRA  ART  LVN  LPN MFCC  FACCP

**Acronyms and metric abbreviations:**

CARE  Project  HOPE  AIDS  mg  mL  L  cm km

**Most abbreviations typed in full capital letters:**

UCLA  PKU  BUN  CMC  COPD  D&C  T&A KSON  CBS

**Abbreviations written in a combination of upper- and lower-case letters:**

Rx  Dx  ACh  Ba  Hb  IgG  mE  q  mOsm  Rh pH  Pap

## 24—2    FRACTIONS

**_DO_**    use a period (decimal point) to separate a decimal fraction from whole numbers, with no spacing before or after the period.

His temperature on admission was 99.9°F.
The new surgical instrument cost $64.85.
The fee for the exam was $85.00. (incorrect)
The fee for the exam was $85. (correct)

## 24—3    INDIRECT QUESTION

**_DO_**    use a period at the end of a request for action that is phrased out of politeness as a question. This places greater emphasis on the requested action.

Would you kindly fill out and return the Medicare form.

Will you please send a copy of the operative report to Dr. Franks.

## 24—4    OUTLINE FIGURES AND NUMBERS

**_DO_**    use a period after a number or letter in an outline or list, and space twice after it. If you desire closure, use a period and double-space after each word or group of words in your outline.

1. Accurate.
2. Grammatically correct.
3. Attractively arranged on the page.

1. Stat duties.   2. Daily responsibilities.
3. Weekly duties.

a. clear,   b. concise,   c. brief,   d. complete.

## 24—5   QUOTATIONS

**DO**    place a period inside quotation marks when the quotation closes the sentence.

The patient related that she spoke with her hands "like an Italian."

## 24—6   REFERENCES

**DO**    use a period to close a bibliographic reference. Haubrich, William S. *Medical Meanings: A Glossary of Word Origins.* San Diego: Harcourt Brace Jovanovich, Inc., 1984.

## 24—7   SENTENCE

**DO**    use a period followed by a double space at the end of a declarative sentence, an imperative sentence, a group of words that express a complete thought, an indirect question, and a footnote.

**Declarative:**
His chest was clear to percussion and auscultation.

**Imperative:**
You must be seen by a surgeon at once.

**A group of words expressing a complete thought:**
Diagnosis:  Myocardial infarction.

**An indirect question:**
Will you please send a copy of the operative report to
Dr. Franks.

**DON'T**   put another period at the end of a sentence that is
closed with an abbreviation that requires a period.

Send this to J. P. Chase and Company Inc.

# 25

# PLURAL

# FORMS

## 25—1    ABBREVIATIONS

***DO***    use an apostrophe to form the plural of lower-case abbreviations and abbreviations that include periods (see Rule 1–14).

M. D.'s   dsg's (dressings)   jt's (joints)

**DON'T**    use an apostrophe with other plural abbreviations.

EKGs   BMRs   TMs   DTRs

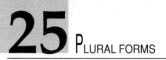

---

## 25—2    BRIEF FORMS

**_DO_**      add an *s* to a brief or short form for a medical term.

bands, segs, monos, lymphs, polys, exams

---

## 25—3    COLLECTIVE NOUNS

**_DO_**      treat a unit of measure as a singular collective noun.

A number of patients **are** having positive reactions.
Forty milliequivalents of KCl **was** given.

---

## 25—4    COMPOUND WORDS

See also Chapter 3, *Apostrophe*.

**_DO_**      add the appropriate plural ending to compound nouns written as one word.

fingerbreadths              teaspoonfuls
spokesmen

**_DO_**      add the appropriate plural ending to the word that is the essential noun in compound nouns written with hyphens or spaces.

chiefs of staff              surgeons general
sisters-in-law

## 25—5    ENGLISH WORDS

**_DO_**    form the plural by adding *s* to the singular word.

myelogram (singular)     myelograms (plural)
disease (singular)       diseases (plural)

**_DO_**    form the plural by adding *es* to nouns that end in *s, x, ch, sh,* or *z.*

stress (singular)        stresses (plural)
helix (singular)         helixes (plural)

patch (singular)         patches (plural)
mash (singular)          mashes (plural)

**_DO_**    form the plural of a noun that ends in *y* preceded by a consonant by changing the *y* to *i* and adding *es.*

mammoplasty (singular)   mammoplasties (plural)
artery (singular)        arteries (plural)

**_DO_**    form the plural of a noun that ends in *o* preceded by a consonant by adding *es* to the singular.

veto (singular)          vetoes (plural)
potato (singular)        potatoes (plural)

**_DO_**    form the plural of most nouns that end in *f* or *fe* by changing the *f* or *fe* to *ves.*

scarf (singular)         scarves (plural)
life (singular)          lives (plural)
calf (singular)          calves (plural)
knife (singular)         knives (plural)

# 25 PLURAL FORMS

## 25—6 EPONYMS

See Rule 25–16.

## 25—7 EXCEPTIONS TO RULES FOR PLURAL ENDINGS

See also Rule 25–17. The words in the following list form plurals in irregular ways:

calyx or calix becomes calyces or calices
comedo becomes comedones
cornu becomes cornua
corpus becomes corpora
femur becomes femora
meatus stays meatus or becomes meatuses
os, which has two meanings, becomes ora for mouths or ossa for
    bones
paries becomes parietes
plexus becomes plexuses
pons becomes pontes
syllabus becomes syllabuses or syllabi
vas becomes vasa
viscus becomes viscera

## 25—8 FRENCH ENDINGS

**_DO_**     form the plural of words that end in _eau_ and _eu_ by
        adding and *x*.

milieu (singular)          milieux (plural)
rouleau (singular)         rouleaux (plural)

## 25—9    GENUS

**DO**    use the plural form of the genus name and if there is no plural form, add the word *organisms* to indicate plural usage.

Streptococcus (singular)    Streptococci (plural)
Trichomonas organisms

## 25—10    GREEK ENDINGS

**DO**    form the plural of words that end in *on* by dropping the *on* and adding an *a*.

criterion (singular)    criteria (plural)
enteron (singular)    entera (plural)
zygion (singular)    zygia (plural)

## 25—11    GREEK OR LATIN ENDINGS

**DO**    form the plural of words that end in *itis* by dropping the *s* and adding *des*.

arthritis (singular)    arthritides (plural)
meningitis (singular)    meningitides (plural)

**DO**    form the plural of words that end in *is* to *es*.

metastasis (singular)    metastases (plural)
diagnosis (singular)    diagnoses (plural)

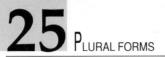

---

## 25—12   ITALIAN ENDINGS

**_DO_**   form the plural of words that end in *o* to by changing the *o* to an *i*.

virtuoso (singular)          virtuosi (plural)

---

## 25—13   LATIN ENDINGS

**_DO_**   form the plural of words that end in *um* by changing the *um* to *a* (pronounced ah).

labium (singular)          labia (plural)

**_DO_**   add an *e* to words that end in *a* (variably pronounced i, e, or a — dictionaries do not agree on pronunciation) to form the plural.

bursa (singular)          bursae (plural)
vertebra (singular)          vertebrae (plural)

**_DO_**   form the plural of words that end in *us* by changing the *us* to *i* (pronounced ī).

alveolus (singular)          alveoli (plural)
meniscus (singular)          menisci (plural)

**_DO_**   form the plural of words that end in *is* by changing the *is* to *es* (pronounced ēs).

anastomosis (singular)          anastomoses (plural)
urinalysis (singular)          urinalyses (plural)

*EXCEPTIONS.*

| | |
|---|---|
| *iris (singular)* | *irides (plural)* |
| *femoris (singular)* | *femora (plural)* |
| *epididymis (singular)* | *epididymides (plural)* |

**_DO_**     form the plural of words that end in *ax* or *ix* by changing the *x* to *c* and adding *es*.

thorax (singular)          thoraces (plural)

**_DO_**     form the plural of words that end in *ex* or *ix* by changing the *ex* or *ix* to *ices*.

appendix (singular)          appendices (plural)
apex (singular)          apices (plural)

**_DO_**     change words that end in *en* by changing the *en* to *ina*.

foramen (singular)          foramina (plural)

**_DO_**     form the plural of words that end in *ma* by changing the *ma* to *mata*.

carcinoma (singular)          carcinomata (plural)

**NOTE.**   *With this ending, it is also permissible to add an s to the singular.*

carcinomas (plural)

**_DO_**     form the plural of words that end in *nx* by changing the *x* to *g* and adding *es*.

phalanx (singular)          phalanges (plural)

**_DO_**  change words that end in _"on"_ by changing the _"on"_ to _a_.

criterion (singular)  criteria (plural)

## 25—14  LETTERS AND ABBREVIATIONS

**_DO_**  use an apostrophe to form the plural of the capital letters A, I, O, M, U and all lower-case single letters (see Rule 3–6).

When you make an entry in the chart, be careful that your 2s don't look like z's.

Spell that with three r's.

You used four I's in the first paragraph.

**_DO_**  use an apostrophe to form the plural of lower-case abbreviations and abbreviations that include periods (see Rule 1–14).

There were elevated wbc's.
It was the M.D.'s decision.

**DON'T**  use the apostrophe to form the plural of numbers or capital letter abbreviations.

The TMs were intact.
There were no 4×4s left in the box.

## 25—15    NUMBERS

**_DO_**     form the plural of figures by adding *s*, but don't use an apostrophe (see Rule 22–18).

1990s
Be sure that your 2s don't look like z's.

**_DO_**     form the plural of written-out numbers just as you form the plural of other words (see Chapter 22, *Numbers*).

She moved here sometime in the forties.

## 25—16    POSSESSIVE NOUNS

**_DO_**     add an apostrophe *s* to plural forms of nouns to show possession (see Rule 3–7).

women's studies
children's ward
mice's tracks

**_DO_**     use an apostrophe after the *s* in plural nouns that end in *s*.

the typists' responsibility (more than one typist)
the Joneses' medical records (more than one Jones)
the heroes' methods
the berries' ripeness
the employees' records

# 25 PLURAL FORMS

**DON'T** use an apostrophe to show possession of institutions or organizations unless they elect to do so.

Veterans Administration Hospital\*      Boys Club
Childrens Hospital      St. Josephs Infirmary

*\*and certainly not Veteran's Hospital!*

**DON'T** use an apostrophe to show possession of eponymic names.

Mueller's saw (incorrect)
Mueller saw (correct)
Penrose's tube (incorrect)
Penrose tube (correct)
The Babinskis showed 3+ on examination. (or 3 plus)

***DO*** show possession with the last noun when two or more nouns share possession (joint possession).

Morgan and Morgan's new patient has just arrived.
Dr. Clark and Dr. Patton's patient was just admitted to the hospital.

**DON'T** use this rule when possession is not shared.

Dr. Clark's and Dr. Patton's patients were just admitted to the hospital.

## 25—17   POSSESSIVE PRONOUNS

See also Rule 26–5.

***DO***  form the possessive of pronouns such as everyone, nobody, someone, anyone, anybody, etc., just as you would with possessive nouns.

It is nobody's fault but your own when you are late for your appointment.

It is anyone's responsibility to enter the prescription refill notation.

It is somebody else's appointment time.

**DON'T**  use an apostrophe with personal pronouns such as its, hers, yours, his, theirs, ours, whose,* or yours.

The next appointment is her's. (incorrect)
The next appointment is hers. (correct)

Dr. Clinton's staff will hold it's quarterly meetings in March, June, September, and December. (incorrect)
Dr. Clinton's staff will hold its quarterly meetings in March, June, September, and December. (correct)

You're coat is soiled. (incorrect)
Your coat is soiled. (correct)

*\*NOTICE THESE CONTRACTIONS, HOWEVER:*

**It's** time for your next appointment.
**Who's** going to clean the operatory?

***COMMENT.***  *Probably one of the most common errors made concerns the misuse of the apostrophe with* it. *Since* its *and* it's *are both correct when used in the proper context, writers often make an improper choice.*

## 25—18    SINGULAR OR PLURAL WORDS

Some medical terms are commonly seen as plurals in all dictation. Because we have two eyes and two ears, physicians commonly dictate the following:

"Conjunctivae are clear."
"Tympanic membranes are intact."

Since heart sounds are multiple, doctors commonly dictate the word *bruits*, which is the plural form of *bruit*. The use of the word determines whether it is singular or plural.

There is no bruit heard.
There are no bruits heard.

Some words can be singular or plural in use.

biceps    triceps    data    facies    series    none    (means *not one* or *not any*)

Some words are always plural in use.

adnexa,    feces,    forceps,    genitalia,    measles, menses,    scabies,    scissors,    tongs,    tweezers

Some words are always singular when used.

ascites    herpes    lues

## 25—19    UNITS OF MEASUREMENT

**_DO_**    use the singular when typing abbreviated units of measurement (cubic centimeters, feet, grams, inches, milligrams, pounds, and so forth).

| | |
|---|---|
| 4 cc | 3 mg |
| 7 ft | 11 lb |
| 10 g | 0.3 in. |
| 5 in. | |

*NOTE.    If you interposed* **of an** *between 0.3 and inch you would not say 0.3 of an inches. This works with any measurement and any decimal part thereof. If the number is one plus a fraction, the sentence should read, "One and one-half inches* **is** *the length of the little finger."* **Note that the verb must be singular.**

**_DO_**    add an *s* to units of measure that are spelled out.

ten centimeters
five milligrams

# P OSSESSIVES

## 26—1   COMPOUND NOUNS

A compound noun consists of two or more distinct words that may be written as one word with a hyphen or hyphens.

**_DO_**    add an *apostrophe s* to the last element of the possessive compound.

the chief-of-staff's decision
my brother-in-law's surgery

## 26—2   EPONYMS

Eponyms are adjectives derived from proper nouns.

**_DO_**    use the rules as stated to form the possessive of eponyms that refer to parts of the anatomy, diseases, signs, or syndromes.

*Signs and Tests:*
Romberg's sign
Hoffmann's reflex
Babinski's sign
Ayer's test

*Anatomy:*
Bartholin's glands
Beale's ganglion
Mauthner's membrane

*Diseases and Syndromes:*
Fallot's tetralogy
Tietze's syndrome
Hirschsprung's disease

**DON'T** show possession for eponyms that describe surgical instruments.

*Instruments:*
Mayo scissors
Richard retractors
Foley catheter
Liston-Stille forceps

**NOTE.** *It is important to note that more and more writers are making exceptions to the possessive rule and not showing the possessive with an eponym. One might expect a change in the rule with more eponyms treated as the eponyms for surgical instruments are treated. In checking dictionaries and other reference books, one finds conflicting spellings: one showing the eponym with the possessive and one showing it without.*

***DO*** when writing for **publication**, substitute the specific descriptive term for a disease for the equivalent eponymic term. Further, if the author prefers the eponym, avoid using the possessive form.

*Preferred:* alopecia parvimaculata syndrome
*Second choice:* Dreuw syndrome
*Not:* Dreuw's syndrome

*Preferred:* pancreatic exocrine insufficiency syndrome
*Second choice:* Clarke-Hadefield syndrome

## 26—3 JOINT POSSESSION

**DO**

show possession with the last noun when two or more nouns share possession.

Clark and Clark's new reference book is in.

Dr. Franklin and Dr. Meadow's patient was just admitted.

**DON'T**

use this rule when possession is not shared.

Dr. Franklin's and Dr. Meadow's **patients were** just admitted.

## 26—4 PLURAL POSSESSIVE NOUNS

**DO**

add an *apostrophe s* ('s) to the plural forms of nouns to show possession.

women's studies
children's ward
mice's tracks

# 26 POSSESSIVES

**_DO_**  use an apostrophe after the *s* in plural nouns that end in *s* to show possession.

the typists' responsibility (more than one typist)
the Joneses' medical records (more than one Jones)
the heroes' methods
the berries' ripeness
the employees' records

**DON'T**  use an apostrophe to show possession of institutions or organizations unless they elect to do so.

Veterans Administration Hospital*
Childrens Hospital
St. Josephs Infirmary
Boys Club

*and certainly not Veteran's Hospital!*

**_DO_**  follow the same rules for forming the possessive of plural abbreviations as for words

It was all the M.D.s' decision.

## 26—5  PRONOUNS

**_DO_**  form the possessive of pronouns such as everyone, nobody, someone, anyone, and anybody, just as you would with possessive nouns.

It is nobody's fault.
That is anyone's guess.
It is somebody else's responsibility.

**DON'T**   use an apostrophe with the personal pronouns such as its,* hers, yours, his, theirs, ours, whose,* or yours.

The next appointment is her's. (incorrect)
The dog injured it's foot. (incorrect)
You're lab coat is soiled. (incorrect)

*NOTICE THESE CONTRACTIONS, HOWEVER*

**It's** time for your next appointment.
**Who's** going to clean the operatory?

**COMMENT.**   *Probably one of the most common errors made concerns the misuse of the apostrophe with* **it**. *Since* its *and* it's *are both correct when used in the proper context, writers often make an improper choice. (See Rule 3–2.)*

## 26—6   SINGULAR POSSESSIVE NOUNS

**_DO_**   use an apostrophe s with a singular noun not ending in s to show possession

the typist's responsibility (one typist)
Bob's doctor
Dr. Mitch's office

**_DO_**   use an apostrophe only (no s) to show possession of singular nouns that end in s or in a strong s sound.

the waitress' table
for appearance' sake
Mr. Gomez' surgery

# 26 POSSESSIVES

**_DO_**   use an apostrophe only after the *s* in two-syllable singular proper nouns ending in *s*.

Frances' report
Mr. Walters' point of view

**DON'T**   break up a proper noun that ends in an *s* by placing the apostrophe in front of the *s*.

*Concerning Mr. Walters:*
Mr. Walter's point of view (incorrect)
Mr. Walters' point of view (correct)

**_DO_**   add an apostrophe *s* to singular nouns ending in *s* or an *s* sound when they are of a single syllable.

Mr. Jones's medical record
James Rose's appointment

## 26—7   TIME, DISTANCE, VALUE, AND SOURCE

**_DO_**   use an apostrophe to show possession of time, distance, value, and source.

return in a month's time
at 10 weeks' gestation
get your money's worth
within a hair's breadth of injury
too much exposure to the sun's rays

**DON'T**   show possession of inanimate things.

the roof of the car *rather than* the car's roof
the color of the bruise *rather than* the bruise's color
the cover of the book *rather than* the book's cover

## 26—8    UNDERSTOOD NOUNS

**_DO_**    follow the same rules for showing possession when the noun is understood.

That stethoscope is Dr. Green's. (stethoscope)
He bought that at William's. (store)

I consulted Dorland's. (dictionary)
That is where he earned his master's. (degree)

# 27

# Progress

## NOTES

## OR CHART

## NOTES

## INTRODUCTION

This chapter gives the do's and don'ts when typing chart notes in a medical practice, since hospital chart notes are usually handwritten progress notes. The information in the patient's chart must always be regarded as confidential.

**_DO_**        transcribe chart notes exactly as dictated. They must be dated and signed or initialed by the dictator, ending with your initials as the typist.

**_DO_**        check daily about the previous day's house calls, emergency calls, and hospital admissions and discharges, so charts can be pulled and entries made.

**DO**     log in every instruction, prescription refills, or telephone call for advice in office medical records.


## 27—1    ABBREVIATIONS

See Chapter 1, *Abbreviations and Symbols*

**DO**     type standard abbreviations and symbols freely into
office chart notes. If hospital chart notes are typed instead of being handwritten, use only those abbreviations approved by the facility.

**DON'T**  use an abbreviation if there is a chance of misinterpretation.

**DO**     type contractions when dictated if the employer approves. Some physicians prefer that contractions be
spelled out.

**DON'T**  abbreviate drug names in chart notes.


## 27—2    ABSTRACTING FROM CHART NOTES

**DO**     abstract information carefully and be extremely accurate when obtaining information from a patient's
medical record to type an insurance claim, letter, or
report. Do NOT guess at abbreviations on the chart.
Be sure you have a release of medical information
form signed by the patient, and give only the information requested.

## 27—3  CONTINUATION PAGES

**_DO_**    type the patient's name on the top of page 2 and on every subsequent page of chart notes.

## 27—4  CONTRACTIONS

**_DO_**    type contractions when dictated if the employer approves. Some physicians prefer that contractions be spelled out.

## 27—5  CORRECTIONS

**_DO_**    draw a line through the error so as not to obliterate the words since a patient's chart is considered a legal document.

**_DO_**    type the correction above or below the error or make a separate correction entry. In the margin, write _correction_ or _Corr._ and your initials if the error is discovered on the same date as typed. If the error is discovered on a subsequent day, be sure to date the error as well as initial it.

**_DO_**    correct errors made while an entry is being typed.

**DON'T**    erase, try to "fix," write over, or type over the error.

**DON'T**    blot out the error with heavy applications of ink or self-adhesive typing strips.

## 27—6    DATES

***DO***      spell out, abbreviate, or type dates in figures. A date
stamp may also be used.

2-4-9x *or* Feb. 4, 199x (preferred)
2/4/9x (acceptable)

## 27—7    DIAGNOSIS (DX) OR IMPRESSION (IMP)

**DON'T**    type an abbreviated diagnosis when dictated, as it is
preferred that diagnoses be spelled out in full. Some
employers allow diagnoses to be abbreviated when
dictated, but an abbreviation can be misinterpreted.

## 27—8    FLAGGING

See Chapter 10, *Editing.*

## 27—9    FORMAT HEADINGS

Some possible headings to use when typing chart
notes follow:

PH (past history) or PMH (past medical history)
Hx (history) or HPI (history of present illness)
CC (chief complaints, signs, or symptoms)
DRUGS
ALLERGIES (allergies to drugs and foods should be
   in capitals and underlined)
PX or PE (physical examination)
VS (vital signs — blood pressure, pulse, respirations,
temperature)
HEENT
LAB, EKG, X-RAYS
CHEST
IMP or DX (impression or diagnosis)
PLAN, RX, or TX (treatment, advice, recommenda-
tion)

The SOAP format headings are as follows:
S — SUBJECTIVE — what the patient tells the
                 physician about the problem.
O — OBJECTIVE — what the physician finds on ex-
                amination.
A — ASSESSMENT — diagnosis based on above.
P — PLAN — what the physician plans — laboratory,
           surgery, medications, referral to another
           doctor, and so forth.

## 27—10   FORMAT STYLES

**_DO_**      single-space and keep margins narrow (not less than
         one-half inch).

**DON'T**   double-space between topics or major headings.

**_DO_**      type main topics in full capitals.

**_DO_**      indent to make topics stand out.

**_DO_** begin each chart note with the date and the patient's name. It is optional to list the patient's birth date and/or age.

Full Block Format (Fig. 27–1)

**_DO_** begin all lines, including headings and subheadings, at the left margin.

**Figure 27–1.** Sample chart entry showing full block format.

Monika M. Takasugi

1-28-9x
CC: Several more episodes of rectal bleeding, always following a BM.
Biopsy and BE essentially negative for source of bleeding.
PE: Anoscopy: moderate hemorrhoidal tags.
Rx: Anusol HC suppositories, 1 morning and evening/6 days. Call or return in 3-4 weeks.

John B. Avery, M. D.
mtf

Indented Style Format (Fig. 27–2)

**_DO_** begin all data single-spaced on the same line as the topic or subtopic.

**_DO_** begin the first and second lines of each paragraph under a major heading two spaces from the heading. Third and subsequent lines should be brought back to the left margin (as long as they clear the outline — if only a few words, block under first two lines).

**Figure 27–2.** Sample chart entry showing indented style format.

---

Philip B. Ward

5-9-9x   HPI: Palpitation. 27 y/o/GII, PII. LMP 4/29/9x
         comes in today for PE. Indicates that is frequently
bothered by feeling of anxiety assoc with palpitations,
has been worked up by previous providers and has been
told is secondary to "nerves."

PMH:    ILL "colitis" in Mex. approx 5 yrs ago. Surg none.
        ALL: Once had abdominal distress after eating
Dungeness crab. MED: None.

PE:     General: Alert 27 y/o/f in NAD. HEENT:
        WNL. Neck: Supple w/o thyromegaly. Chest:
Clear. COR S1, S2 normal w/o murmurs. Breast: Benign.
Abdomen: Soft nontender. Bowel sounds present w/o
organomegaly. Back: Straight, nontender. Pelvic: Ext.
WNL. VAG: w/o lesions. CX: Benign. UT: WNL in mid-
line. Extremities: w/o lesions. Neuro: Oriented x 3.
Motor: Good symmetrical strength of all extremities.
Sensory: Intact. COOR: Good. CN II-XII* intact. DTRs +2.

Dx:     1. Anxiety state with hyperventilation syn-
           drome.
        2. Palpitation most likely secondary to #1.
        3. Hx of irritable bowel syndrome, currently
           stable.

Tx:     Advised on brown paper bag use, dimension
        reflex 2, RTC 1 mo for f/u.


                        _____
                        Byron T. O'Connor, M. D.
mtf

---

* Optional: CN 2-12 would be typed if Roman numerals were not
available in the fonts on the computer software.

Modified Block Style Format (Fig. 27–3)

**_DO_**     indent subtopics 3 to 5 spaces under the main topics.

**_DO_**     begin all data single-spaced on the same line as the
            topic or subtopic. Tabulate over from the left margin.

**Figure 27–3.**   Sample chart entry showing modified block style.

| | |
|---|---|
| Tammy O. Beckley | BD: 02-15-89 |
| | Age: 1 |
| | |
| 5-1-9x | Sunday, 3 a.m., pt seen in ER complain-ing of pain, a.d./3 days. PX revealed fluid and pus. |
| | Temp 101. |
| ADVICE: | Myringotomy. |
| IMPRESSION: | Rt otitis media. |
| | |
| | _____ |
| | Kathleen F. King, M. D. |
| mtf | |

SOAP Style Format

See Figure 27–4 for a sample of the SOAP style format.

**Figure 27–4.** Sample chart entry showing SOAP (Subjective, Objective, Assessment, Plan) method.

---

Vincent M. Liu

10-11-9x

S: Epigastric pain. Improved with diet. Plan previously described.
O: Abdomen: Benign.
A: Epigastric discomfort improved; obesity.
P: Cont 1200 ADA diet. RTC in 3 mo for f/u or sooner p.r.n.

 _____
 Lewis V. Franklin, M. D.

mtf

---

## 27—11 HANDWRITTEN ENTRIES

*DO* abstract accurately. Any entry that is questionable as to its interpretation should be verified by the physician. Some examples of misinterpretations follow:

NBM can mean no bowel movement or normal bowel movement depending on which hospital you are working in.

U (units) can be mistaken for a zero (0) i.e., 6 U of insulin can be mistaken for 60 units of insulin. Units should always be written out in chart notes.

OD can mean right eye or medication to be taken once daily.

q.d. (once a day) has been misinterpreted as q.i.d. (4 times daily).

C, MS, and CF have more than 10 possible meanings each.

**_DO_**     verify with the physician any abbreviated drug names. Here are just a few of the many examples of misinterpretations.

CPZ (Compazine or chlorpromazine)

PBZ (phenylbutazone, pyribenzamine, or phenoxylbenzamine)

HCT250 (hydrocortisone) was misinterpreted as HCTZ50 (hydrochlorothiazide)

## 27—12    HISTORY AND PHYSICAL

See also Chapter 14, *History and Physical Format.* Some chart notes can be a formal history and physical report to an attorney, a worker's compensation insurance company, or a referring physician (consultation report).

**_DO_**     place an entry in the medical record if the physician dictates a document.

2-7-9x  See note to Dr. Normington.

mlo

*also correct*
Feb. 7, 199x  See note to Dr. Normington.                mlo

## 27—13    INFORMATION OR DATA SHEET

**_DO_**        transfer all of the appropriate patient information to the initial page of the medical record.

## 27—14    MEDICATION

**_DO_**        underline and type in full capitals drug and food allergies.

**_DO_**        spell out all drug names.

**_DO_**        make entries for refill prescriptions given via telephone.

## 27—15    NUMBERS

See Chapter 22, *Numbers.*

## 27—16    PHYSICAL EXAMINATION (PX OR PE)

See Chapter 14, *History and Physical Format*, Rule 14—4 for headings.

## 27—17    PRESSURE SENSITIVE PAPER

**DON'T**    use pressure sensitive paper to correct or obliterate chart notes.

## 27—18    SIGNATURE LINE

**_DO_**    type a signature line or leave adequate space for the dictator's signature or initials.

## 27—19    TELEPHONE

**_DO_**    make entries in regard to telephone advice.

**_DO_**    make entries for prescription refills via telephone.

# 28

# PROOFREADING

# AND

# REVISIONS

## INTRODUCTION

Proofread your work carefully. Accuracy is important in spelling, grammar, figures, word division, and punctuation. Professional quality is demanded in all medical reports. The importance of errors varies of course. For example, transposed letters in the name of a drug could be very serious, whereas variations in a format and style may be acceptable. Equipment limitations are never an excuse for less than professional quality copy. Please refer to Figure 28–1 for the symbols used in proofreading and what they mean.

## 28—1   ABBREVIATIONS, SYMBOLS, AND NUMBERS

**DO**        know the technical symbols in your specialty area. Avoid the use of abbreviations in records where they are inappropriate. See Chapter 1 for help with abbreviations, Chapter 22 for help with numbers.

| Mark | Explanation | Example | Result |
|---|---|---|---|
| ¶ | paragraph | ... high fever. On physical exam ... | ... high fever. |
| no ¶ | no paragraph | On physical exam I found a | ... high fever. On physical exam ... |
| ⊙ | change to period | ... high fever On physical exam ... | ... high fever. On physical exam ... |
| < | insert | Your patient came in to see me | Your patient came in to see me |
| ⊙ | insert semicolon | blood pressure: 130/90 temperature | blood pressure: 130/90; temperature |
| ʼ | insert apostrophe | She doesnt remember asking for | She doesn't remember asking for |
| ( ) | insert parentheses | (1)Sterile field. (2)Suture materials | (1) Sterile field. (2) Suture materials |
| = | insert hyphen | She was seen in follow up exam on | She was seen in follow-up exam on |
| ⌃ | insert comma | Jean Brun your patient, came in | Jean Brun, your patient, came in |
| ⊙ | insert colon | Diagnosis Appendicitis | Diagnosis: Appendicitis |
| ˇ | insert quotation marks | There has been some hurting in my | There has been some "hurting" in my |
| ][ | center | ]Physical Examination[ | Physical Examination |
| cap ≡ | use capital letters | Physical Examination | PHYSICAL EXAMINATION |
| | don't spell out | There was fifty-seven cents | There was 57 cents |

| Mark | Explanation | Example | Result |
|------|-------------|---------|--------|
| ? | is this correct? | I saw your patient Janeé Brun | I saw your patient Jane Brun |
| ℓ or ⎯ | delete | Jean Brun, ~~your patient~~, came in | Jean Brun came in |
| / | delete or change | Jean Brun, your patient, came in | Jean Brun, your patient, came in |
| # | space | JeanBrun, your patient, came in | Jean Brun, your patient, came in |
| ∼ | transpose | Jean Brun, your patient, came in | Your patient Jean Brun came in |
| ( ) | close up space | Jean Brun, your patient, came in | Jean Brun, your patient, came in |
| stet... | let it alone | Jean Brun, your patient, came in | Jean Brun, your patient, came in |
| ⌐ | move left | Jean Brun, your patient, came in | |
| ⌐ | move right | Jean Brun, your patient, came in | |
| [ | move up | Jean Brun, your patient, came in | |
| ] | move down | Jean Brun, your patient, came in | |
| ℓc or / | use lower case | Jean Brun, your patient, came in | Jean Brun, your patient, came in |
| ∼ | delete and close | I can see its surface now | I can see its surface now |
| ○ | spell out | There were 2 patients to be | There were two patients to be |

**Figure 28–1.** Proofreading marks with explanations.

# 28 PROOFREADING AND REVISIONS

## 28—2 CAPITALIZATION

**_DO_** know why you are using a capital letter. When in doubt, always take the time to check on a rule or look for the word in a reference book. See Chapter 4 for help with any capitalization problem that you may have.

## 28—3 FLAGGING

**DON'T** type material that does not make sense to you. If you cannot understand a word and the dictator is un-available, leave a blank space in your material that is long enough to allow you to insert the correct word later. Attach a flag sheet to the material. This flagging (also called carding, tagging, or marking) can best be done by using the repositionable adhesive notes. You can also staple or paper clip your card or flag. The flag should include the patient's name, the page number, the paragraph, and the line of the missing word. If you are in a large organization, add your name. It will help the dictator if you put the missing word(s) in context, that is, include a few words that come before and after it. An example of a flag follows:

Williams, Maribeth #18-74-78. Under PX, CR.
(page 2, line 8) "_____? respirations present."
Sounds like "chain smokes." Judy, 5-17-91
(The dictator will return a note that reads "Cheyne-Stokes respirations present.")

(See Figure 10–1, page 106.)

## 28—4   PROOFREADING

**_DO_**   proofread carefully and correct all errors. Double-check any vital materials you have transcribed. When there is any doubt about the material, flag the work for the dictator's attention. Mistakes tend to cluster. If you find one typo, look carefully for another one nearby.

**_DO_**   learn where you generally make errors and check these areas first. Read everything in the copy straight through from beginning to end: titles, subtitles, punctuation, capitalization, indented items, and page numbers.

**_DO_**   put your copy aside for a break before checking it. It is also helpful to work on another project and alternate proofreading and production.

**_DO_**   read the pages of a long document out of order.

**_DO_**   read your copy backwards when checking for spelling errors. Read your copy out loud to check for punctuation errors.

**_DO_**   double-check references such as "see the chart below."

**_DO_**   check figures aloud with a partner. Double-check proper column placement and look for misplaced commas and decimal points.

**DO** scrutinize features that come in sets, such as brackets, parentheses, quotation marks, and dashes.

**DON'T** proofread your own copy. Trade transcripts with someone unfamiliar with the material but familiar with the general topic.

**DO** double-check a final draft after printing out your corrected copy. Often the changes in a document will affect the printout in unexpected ways: the last line appearing alone on the final page; one parenthesis or bracket being printed on the line following; a number being separated from the symbol following it; page numbers being changed inappropriately; long spaces appearing between words or figures; indenting appearing inconsistently; type fonts, italics, underlining, superscript, or boldface printing out inappropriately.

## 28—5 PUNCTUATION

**DO** know why you are using a particular punctuation mark. Remember that leaving out required punctuation is as much an error as putting in an unneeded mark or using the wrong mark. Review the rules from time to time and refer to the chapters in this book for guidance when you need it.

## 28—6 REVISIONS AND CORRECTIONS ON THE TYPEWRITER

**DO** Try to make your corrections so that your copy will not have to be retyped. Use good correction tools: a soft brush, correction fluid, correction tape, lift-off tape with correctable film ribbon.

**_DO_**      try to realign material properly in the typewriter and use typewriter functions to make corrections (when this is available).

**DON'T**      attempt to cover up large mistakes with correction fluid unless you are making a master for photocopy material. (Correction fluid is best saved for punctuation errors.)

**DON'T**      use an eraser over a keyboard.

**DON'T**      place paper with wet correction fluid back under the platen in a typewriter.

**DON'T**      use correction tape unless you are making a master for photocopy material.

## 28—7    ROUGH DRAFT

**_DO_**      double space rough draft material that is intended for revision or editing.

## 28—8    SPELLING

**_DO_**      consult a dictionary, speller, or word book whenever you have the slightest doubt about your spelling.

## 28—9    WORD DIVISION

**_DO_**    divide words only at the proper point when you must divide a word. Consult a word book for assistance when you are in doubt about word division. See Chapter 15, _Hyphen Use and Word Division,_ for help.

# 29

# QUESTION

# MARK

---

## 29—1   DASHES

**_DO_**     use dashes to set off a parenthetical question within a sentence. Place the question mark before the closing dash.

The pharmaceutical representative from Burroughs Wellcome — do you know her? — has she called again for an appointment?

**_DO_**     use a question mark to end an interrogative phrase following a closing dash.

Is the medical convention in Hawaii? — on Maui?

## 29—2 PARENTHESES

**DON'T** use a question mark before the closing parenthesis unless it refers to the parenthetical item or the sentence ends with a different mark of punctuation.

Can you send me a copy of the pathology report (and can you send me two?), or must I request it in writing?

The patient's name is Mary Barker (or is it Merry Parker?).

*DO* use a question mark outside the closing parenthesis if the phrase in parentheses is to be incorporated at the end of a sentence.

Do you know Barry Smith (or is it Berry Smyth)?

Please order a CBC on Mrs. Warren (can the lab send me four copies of the report?), and I must have the results by Friday.

## 29—3 PUNCTUATION

*DO* use a question mark at the end of a sentence to indicate a direct question.

*NOTE. Leave two spaces after a question mark before typing the next sentence.*

When will Mr. Hamlin have the gallbladder surgery?

*DO* use question marks to indicate a series of questions pertaining to the same subject and verb.

*NOTE. Leave only one space after a question mark within a sentence.*

Shall I send the report to Dr. Jones? Dr. Keystone? Dr. Avery?

***DO*** use a question mark to show doubt.

The complete blood count showed 20,000 (?) white blood cells.

## 29—4   QUOTATION MARKS

***DO*** type a question mark outside a closing quotation mark if the entire sentence is in the form of a question.

Will you answer my question, "What year were you born"?

***DO*** type a question mark inside a closing quotation mark if only the quoted material is a question.

The medical report answers my original question, "What is the secondary diagnosis?"

***DO*** use quotation marks outside the closing question mark when a quoted sentence stands alone or is at the beginning or end of a sentence.

"Can you dictate the report on Mr. Bowen right now?" she asked.

## 29—5    SPACING

**_DO_**        use two spaces after a question mark at the end of a
sentence.

> **NOTE.**   *There is no space after a question mark when
> another mark of punctuation (closing quotation mark,
> parenthesis, or dash) immediately follows.*

# 30

## QUOTATION

## MARKS

## 30—1 EXACT WORDS

**_DO_**    use quotation marks to enclose the **exact** words of a speaker.

The patient said, "There has been hurting in the pelvis bones."
The patient said that there had been some pain in the pelvis.

The patient said he's always felt like "something's hung up in there." (Note where the quotes begin.)
The patient said "he's always felt like something's hung up in there." (Incorrect. Patient would not say "he's always felt . . . ")

## 30—2   PUNCTUATION WITH QUOTATION MARKS

**_DO_**   place periods and commas **inside** the closing quotation mark; semicolons and colons **outside** the closing quotation mark.

The tenth chapter, "Editing," is the most difficult for me.

The patient related that she spoke with her hands "like an Italian."

**_DO_**   place a question mark or an exclamation point inside the closing quotation marks when it applies to the material quoted and outside when it applies to the entire sentence.

Dr. Matthews exclaimed, "I must return to the Coronary Care Unit at once!"

Patients often ask, "When can I return to work?"

**_DO_**   use a colon to introduce quoted material if the introductory material is an independent clause.

Patients often ask me this: "When can I return to work?"

**_DO_**   use a comma to introduce quoted material unless the quotation is part of the flow of the sentence.

Her favorite response is that "we've always done it this way."

The patient stated, "a roll of paper fell and struck me across the upper back and knocked me to the ground."

## 30—3  SPECIAL ATTENTION

***DO***    use quotation marks to enclose single words or phrases for special attention.

I can see no need for "temper tantrums" in the operating suite.

The German expression "Gemütlichkeit" exactly described the feelings we had during your father's visit.

***DO***    use quotation marks to enclose slang, coined, awkward, whimsical, or humorous words that might show ignorance on the part of the writer if it is not known that he/she is aware of them.

See if you can schedule a few "well" patients for a change.

Some of the expressions that startle the novice transcriptionist are "pink puffer" and "blue bloater."

If you have "clergyman's knee," "tailor's seat," "tennis elbow," or "trigger finger," what you really have is a form of bursitis or tendinitis.

## 30—4  TITLES

***DO***    place titles of minor literary works within quotation marks.

His photographic entry "The Country Doctor" won first place in the contest.

# 30

**_DO_**   place titles of chapters, sections, and other sub-
divisions of a published work within quotation
marks. (The titles of published books, magazines, and
articles are underlined.) See Rule 4–17 for proper
capitalization of literary works.

Your homework assignment is to read "Capitalization" in <u>Medical Typing and Transcribing: Techniques
and Procedures</u>.

# 31

R EFERENCE

MATERIALS

AND

PUBLICATIONS

# 31 REFERENCE MATERIALS AND PUBLICATIONS

## 31—1 ABBREVIATIONS DICTIONARIES — GENERAL

Crowley, Ellen T., and Helen E. Sheppard (eds.), *Reverse International Acronyms, Initialisms, and Abbreviations Dictionary*, Detroit, Gale Research Company, 1985.

Paxton, John (ed.), *Everyman's Dictionary of Abbreviations*, Totowa, N.J., B & N Imports, 1986.

Spillner, Paul, *World Guide to Abbreviations*, vols. 1–3, ed. 2, New York, R.R. Bowker, 1973.

## 31—2 ABBREVIATIONS DICTIONARIES — MEDICAL

*The Charles Press Handbook of Current Medical Abbreviations*, Philadelphia, The Charles Press Publishers, 1985.

Davis, Neil M., *Medical Abbreviations: 4200 Conveniences at the Expense of Communications and Safety*, Huntingdon Valley, PA, Neil M. Davis Associates, 1987.

Delong, Marilyn Fuller, *Medical Acronyms and Abbreviations*. Oradell, NJ, Medical Economics Books, 1989.

Garb, Solomon, et al., *Abbreviations and Acronyms in Medicine and Nursing*. New York, Springer Publishing Company, 1976.

Hughes, Harold K., *Dictionary of Abbreviations in Medicine and Health Sciences*, Lexington, MA, Health, 1977.

Jablonski, Stanley, *Dictionary of Medical Acronyms and Abbreviations*, St. Louis, MO, The C. V. Mosby Company, 1987.

Keller, J.J., *The Modernized Metric System Explained*, Neenah, WI, J. J. Keller and Associates, 1974.

Kerr, Avice, *Medical Hieroglyphs, Abbreviations and Symbols*, Downey, CA, Enterprise Publications, 1970.

Logan, Carolynn and M. Katherine Rice, *Logan's Medical and Scientific Abbreviations*, Philadelphia, J. B. Lippincott Company, 1987.

*Medical Abbreviations: A Cross Reference Dictionary*, Lansing, MI, The Special Studies Committee of the Michigan Occupational Therapy Association, 1977.

*Medical Abbreviations Handbook*, Oradell, NJ, Medical Economics, 1983.

*Quick Directory of Medical Abbreviations*, Darien, CT, Miller and Fink Corporation, 1977.

Roody, Peter, et al., *Medical Abbreviations and Acronyms,* New York, McGraw-Hill Book Company, 1977.

Schertel, A., *Abbreviations in Medicine,* New York, S. Karger, 1984.

Sloane, Sheila B., *Medical Abbreviations and Eponyms,* Philadelphia, W. B. Saunders Company, 1985.

Sloane, Sheila B., *The Medical Word Book,* Philadelphia, W. B. Saunders Company, 1982.

Steen, Edwin B., *Medical Abbreviations,* ed. 5., Philadelphia, W. B. Saunders Company, 1984.

*Stylebook/Editorial Manual of the AMA,* Littleton, MS, Publishing Sciences Group, 1976.

Venolia, Jan, *Write Right!,* Woodland Hills, CA, Periwinkle Press, 1980.

## 31—3  ANTONYMS, EPONYMS, HOMONYMS, SYNDROMES, AND SYNONYMS

Chapman, Robert L., *Roget's International Thesaurus,* ed 4., New York, Harper & Row, 1984.

Fernald, James C., *English Synonyms and Antonyms with Notes on the Correct Use of Prepositions,* Darby, PA, Arden Library, 1981.

Magalini, Sergio I., *Dictionary of Medical Syndromes,* ed. 2., Philadelphia, J. B. Lippincott Company, 1981.

Rodale, J. I., *The Synonym Finder,* Emmaus, PA, Rodale Press, 1978.

*Webster's New Dictionary of Synonyms,* Springfield, MA, G & C Merriam Company, 1973.

*Webster's Synonyms, Antonyms, and Homonyms,* Alhambra, CA, Dennison, 1974.

## 31—4  CAREER DEVELOPMENT

*American Association for Medical Transcription Journal,* Modesto, CA, American Association for Medical Transcription, quarterly.

*American Association for Medical Transcription Newsletter,* Modesto, CA, American Association for Medical Transcription, bi-monthly.

*Analysis: Civil Service Classification of Medical Transcriptionist,* Modesto, CA, American Association for Medical Transcription, 1981.

Dennis, Robert Lee, and Jean Monty Doyle, *The Complete Handbook for Medical Secretaries and Assistants,* Boston, Little, Brown and Company, 1978.

Fordney, Marilyn T. and Joan M. Follis, *Administrative Medical Assisting,* New York, John Wiley and Sons, 1989.

Health Professions Institute, *Perspectives on the Medical Transcription Profession,* Modesto, CA, 1988.

Kinn, Mary E., *The Administrative Medical Assistant,* Philadelphia, W. B. Saunders Company, 1988.

## 31—5    CERTIFICATION

*The AAMT Test Guide,* Modesto, CA, American Association for Medical Transcription, 1982.

## 31—6    COMPOSITION

Andrews, William D. and Deborah C. Andrews, *Write For Results,* Boston, Little Brown and Company, 1982.

Blumenthal, Lassor A., *Successful Business Writing,* New York, Putnam Publishing Group, 1985.

Brogan, John A., *Clear Technical Writing,* New York, McGraw-Hill Book Company, 1973.

*Funk and Wagnalls Standard Desk Dictionary,* New York, Harper & Row, 1984.

Hodges, John C. and Mary E. Whitten (eds.), *Harbrace College Handbook,* ed. 8., New York, Harcourt, Brace, Jovanovich, 1984.

*Random House Dictionary of the English Language,* New York, Random House, 1987.

Ross-Larson, Bruce, *Edit Yourself — A Manual for Everyone Who Works with Words,* New York, W. W. Norton and Company, 1982.

*Secretary's Portfolio of Letters Most Often Used in a Physician's Office,* West Nyack, NY, Parker Publishing Company, 1968.

Skillin, Marjorie E. and Robert M. Gay, *Words into Type,* Englewood Cliffs, NJ, Prentice-Hall, 1974.

## 31—7    EDITING

Plotnik, Arthur, *The Elements of Editing*, Macmillan Publishing Company, New York, 1982.

## 31—8    ENGLISH HANDBOOKS (GRAMMAR, PUNCTUATION, AND GENERAL CLERICAL INFORMATION)

Branchaw, Bernadine P. and Bowman, Joel P., *SRA Reference Manual for Office Personnel*, Chicago, SRA Science Research Associates, 1986.

Clark, James L. and Lyn Clark, *How 4: A Handbook for Office Workers*, Belmont, CA, Kent Publishing Company, 1985.

Flesch, Rudolf, *Look It Up*, New York, Harper & Row, 1977.

Hodges, John C., *Harbrace College Handbook*, Harcourt, Brace, Jovanovich, Orlando, FL, 1986.

House, Clifford R. and Kathie Sigler, *Reference Manual for Office Personnel*, Cincinnati, South Western Publishing Company, 1981.

Irmscher, W. F., *The Holt Guide to English: A Comprehensive Handbook of Rhetoric, Language, and Literature*, New York, Holt, Rinehart and Winston, 1981.

Johnson, Edward, *Handbook of Good English*, New York, Facts on File Publisher, 1983.

Klein, A. E., *The New World Secretarial Handbook*, Cleveland, William Collins-World Publishing Company, 1973.

Longyear, Marie M., *The McGraw-Hill Style Manual: Concise Guide for Writers and Editors*, New York, McGraw-Hill Book Company, 1982.

Perrin, P. G. and J. W. Corder, *Handbook of Current English*, Glenview, IL, Scott Foresman and Company, 1975.

Sabin, William A., *The Gregg Reference Manual*, New York, McGraw-Hill Book Company, 1985.

Shaw, Harry, *Punctuate It Right!*, New York, Harper & Row, 1986.

Shertzer, Margaret D., *The Elements of Grammar*, New York, Macmillan Publishing Company, 1986.

Strumpf, Michael, and Auriel Douglas, *Painless Perfect Grammar*, New York, Monarch Press, 1985.

*Stylebook/Editorial Manual of the American Medical Association*, Littleton, MS, Publishing Sciences Group, 1976.

# 31 REFERENCE MATERIALS AND PUBLICATIONS

## 31—9 EPONYMS

See Rule 31–3.

## 31—10 HOMONYMS

See Rule 31–3.

## 31—11 HUMOR AND GAMES FOR MEDICAL TYPISTS AND TRANSCRIPTIONISTS

Pitman, Sally C. (ed.), *The eMpTy Laugh Book,* Modesto, CA, American Association for Medical Transcription, 1981.

Tank, Hazel (ed.), *The Puzzlement for Medical Transcriptionists,* Modesto, CA, American Association for Medical Transcription, 1981.

## 31—12 INSURANCE

Fordney, Marilyn T., *Insurance Handbook for the Medical Office,* ed. 3., Philadelphia, W. B. Saunders Company, 1989.

## 31—13 LAW AND ETHICS

American Medical Association, *Judicial Council Opinions and Reports,* Chicago, American Medical Association, 1976.

American Medical Association, *Medicolegal Forms with Legal Analysis,* Chicago, American Medical Association, 1973.

Bander, Edward J. and Jeffrey J. Wallach, *Medical Legal Dictionary,* Dobbs Ferry, NY, Oceana Publications, 1970.

Black, Henry Campbell, *Black's Law Dictionary,* St. Paul, MN, West Publishing Company, 1979.

Brody, Howard, *Ethical Decisions in Medicine,* Boston, Little, Brown and Company, 1981.

Ehrlich, Ann, *Ethics and Jurisprudence,* Champaign, IL, The Colwell Company, 1983.

Flight, Myrtle R., *Law, Liability, and Ethics for Medical Office Personnel,* Albany, New York, Delmar Publishers, Inc., 1988.

Hayt, Emanuel, *Medicolegal Aspects of Hospital Records,*Berwyn, IL, Physician's Record Company, 1977.

Heller, Marjorie K., *Legal P's and Q's in the Doctor's Office,* Bayside, NY, Lawyer's Bookshelf, 1981.

Holder, Angela Roddey, *Medical Malpractice Law,* New York, John Wiley and Sons, 1978.

Huffman, Edna K., *Medical Record Management,* Berwyn, IL, Physician's Record Company, 1985.

Kapp, Marshall B., *Legal Guide for Medical Office Managers,* Chicago, IL, Pluribus Press, Inc., 1985.

Lewis, Marcia A. and Carol D. Warden, *Law and Ethics in the Medical Office Including Bioethical Issues,* ed. 2., Philadelphia, F. A. Davis Company, 1988.

Scott, Walter L., *Medicolegal Glossary,* Oradell, NJ, Medical Economics, 1989.

## 31—14    MEDICAL DICTIONARIES

*Blakiston's Gould Medical Dictionary* New York, McGraw-Hill Book Company, 1979.

Critchley, Macdonald, *Butterworth's Medical Dictionary,* Woburn, MA, Butterworth Publishers, 1980.

*Dorland's Illustrated Medical Dictionary,* ed. 27., Philadelphia, W. B. Saunders Company, 1988.

Franks, Richard and H. Swartz, *Simplified Medical Dictionary,* Oradell, NJ, Medical Economics, 1977.

*Glossary of Hospital Terms,* Chicago, American Medical Record Association, 1974.

Gomez, Joan, *Dictionary of Symptoms,* Briarcliff Manor, NY, Stein & Day, 1983.

Hinsie, Leland E. and Robert J. Campbell, *Psychiatric Dictionary,* New York, Oxford University Press, 1970.

Isler, Charlotte, *Isler's Pocket Dictionary: A Guide to Disorders and Diagnostic Tests,* Oradell, NJ, Medical Economics, 1984.

Melloni, Biagio John, and Gilbert M. Eisner, *Melloni's Illustrated Medical Dictionary,* Baltimore, The Williams and Wilkins Company, 1985.

Miller, Benjamin F. and Claire B. Keane, *Encyclopedia and Dictionary of Medicine, Nursing and Allied Health,* ed. 3., Philadelphia, W. B. Saunders Company, 1983.

Pyle, Vera, *Current Medical Terminology,* Modesto, CA, Prima Vera Publications, 1988.

Scott, Walter L., *Medicolegal Glossary,* Oradell, NJ, Medical Economics, 1989.

*Stedman's Medical Dictionary,* Baltimore, The Williams and Wilkins Company, 1981.

Thomas, Clayton L. (ed.), *Taber's Cyclopedic Medical Dictionary,* Philadelphia, F. A. Davis Company, 1985.

Urdang, Laurence, and Helen H. Swallow, *Mosby's Medical and Nursing Dictionary,* St. Louis, C. V. Mosby Company, 1986.

Wakeley, Sir Cecil, *The Farber Medical Dictionary.,* Philadelphia, J. B. Lippincott Company, 1975.

White, Wallace F., *Language of the Health Sciences,* New York, John Wiley and Sons, 1977.

## 31—15   MEDICAL RECORDS

Gordon, B. L., *Simplified Medical Records System,* Acton, MA, Publishing Sciences Group, 1975.

*Hospital Medical Records: Guidelines for Their Use and Release of Medical Information,* Chicago, American Medical Association, 1972.

*Medical Record Departments in Hospitals: Guide to Organization,* Chicago, American Hospital Association, 1972.

Mosier, Alice, and Frank J. Pace, *Medical Records Technology,* Indianapolis, IN, Bobbs-Merrill Company, 1975.

## 31—16    MEDICAL TERMINOLOGY

Austrin, Miriam G., *Young's Learning Medical Terminology Step by Step*, St. Louis, C. V. Mosby Company, 1983.

Bradbury, Peggy F., *Transcriber's Guide to Medical Terminology*, Garden City, NY, Medical Examination Publishing Company, 1973.

Chabner, Davi-Ellen, *The Language of Medicine, A Write-In Text Explaining Medical Terms*, Philadelphia, W. B. Saunders Company, 1985. (cassettes available)

Cohen, Alan Y., *Medicine/Biology Terminology Cards* (1,000 flash cards), Springfield, OH, Visual Education Association, 1978.

DeLorenzo, Barbara, and Doris Fedun, *Medical Terminology*, Vol. I, A–I and Vol. II, M–Z, Thorofare, NJ, Slack, 1988.

Dunmore, Charles W. and Rita M. Fleischer, *Medical Terminology: Exercises in Etymology*, Philadelphia, F. A. Davis Company, 1985.

Fisher, J. Patrick, *Basic Medical Terminology*, Indianapolis, IN, Bobbs-Merrill Company, 1983. (cassettes available)

Frenay, Sister Agnes, *Understanding Medical Terminology*, Haverford, PA, Catholic Hospital Association, 1984. (transparencies available)

Gross, Verlee E., *Mastering Medical Terminology: Textbook of Anatomy, Diseases, Anomalies and Surgeries with English Translation and Pronunciation*, Simi Valley, CA, Halls of Ivy Press, 1969.

Gross, Verlee E., *The Structure of Medical Terms*, Simi Valley, CA, Halls of Ivy Press, 1973.

Kinn, Mary E., *Medical Terminology Review Challenge*, Albany, NY, Delmar Publishers, 1987.

LaFleur, Myrna Weber, and Winifred K. Starr, *Exploring Medical Language*, St. Louis, C. V. Mosby Company, 1985. (computer software available)

Leonard, Peggy, *Building a Medical Vocabulary*, Philadelphia, W. B. Saunders Company, 1988 (cassettes and computer software available)

Prendergast, Alice, *Medical Terminology: A Text/Workbook*, Reading, MA, Addison-Wesley Publishing Company, 1983.

Smith, Genevieve Love, and Phyllis E. Davis, *Medical Terminology, A Programmed Text*, New York, John Wiley and Sons, 1981. (cassettes available).

Sormunen, Carolee, *Terminology for Allied Health Professionals*, Cincinnati, OH, South-Western Publishing Company, 1985. (cassettes available).

Sorrells, Sally (Ingmire), Medical Vocabulary from A to Z. Mountain View, CA, Western Tape, 1981. (cassettes available)

Wroble, Eugene M., *Terminology for the Health Professions*, Philadelphia, J. B. Lippincott Company, 1982.

## 31—17    MEDICAL TERMINOLOGY GUIDES

*Current Procedural Terminology,* Chicago, American Medical Association, 1977.

Rimer, Evelyn H., *Harbeck's Glossary of Medical Terms.*, Brisbane, CA, San Francisco, WEB Offset, 1967.

Stegeman, Wilson, *Medical Terms Simplified,* St. Paul, MN, West Publishing Company, 1975.

Strand, Helen R., *An Illustrated Guide to Medical Terminology,* Baltimore, The Williams and Wilkins Company, 1968.

## 31—18    PHARMACEUTICAL

Beebe, Judy, *Instant Drug Index,* Palo Alto, CA, William Kaufmann. (updates available spring and fall of each year)

Billups, Norman F., *American Drug Index,* Philadelphia, J. B. Lippincott Company. (annual publication)

DeLorenzo, Barbara, *Pharmaceutical Terminology,* Thorofare, NJ, Slack, 1988.

Griffith, H. Winter, M. D., *Complete Guide to Prescription and Nonprescription Drugs.* Tucson, AZ, H. P. Books, Inc., 1987.

*Hospital Formulary.* Washington, D.C., American Society of Hospital Pharmacists, 1978.

Kastrup, Erwin K. and Bernie R. Olin, III, *Facts and Comparisons,* Philadelphia, J. B. Lippincott Company (updated monthly)

Lewis, Arthur J., *Modern Drug Encyclopedia and Therapeutic Index,* New York, The Yorke Medical Group, The Dun-Donnelly Publishing Corporation, 1973.

*Medi-Spell Transcriber's Bulletin,* P. O. Box 2546, Mission Viejo, CA 92690. (published quarterly list of current drugs)

*National Drug Code Directory,* Volumes 1 and 2, Washington, D.C., U.S. Government Printing Office, 1980.

*National Formulary XIV* (N.F.), Washington, D.C., American Pharmaceutical Association, 1975.

Patterson, H. Robert, Edward A. Gustafson, and Eleanor Sheridan, *Falconer's Current Drug Handbook,* Philadelphia, W. B. Saunders Company, 1984–1986.

*Physicians' Desk Reference for Nonprescription Drugs,* Oradell, NJ, Medical Economics. (annual publication)

*Physicians' Desk Reference for Ophthalmology,* Oradell, NJ, Medical Economics. (annual publication)

*Physicians' Desk Reference: The Indices,* Oradell, NJ, Medical Economics. (annual publication)

*Physicians' Desk Reference to Pharmaceutical Specialties and Biologists (PDR),* Oradell, NJ, Medical Economics. (annual publication)

*Physicians' Desk Reference for Radiology and Nuclear Medicine,* Oradell, NJ, Medical Economics. (annual publication)

Shirkey, Harry C., *Pediatric Dosage Handbook,* Washington, D.C., American Pharmaceutical Association, 1980.

Squire, Jessie E. and Jean M. Welch, *Basic Pharmacology for Nurses,* St. Louis, C. V. Mosby Company, 1977.

Turley, Susan M., *Understanding Pharmacology,* Modesto, CA, Health Professions Institute, 1988.

*The United States Pharmacopoeia* (U.S.P.), Rockville, MD, The Pharmacopoeia of the United States of America, 1984. (annual supplements)

## 31—19    PROOFREADING

Dewar, Thadys J. and H. Frances Daniels, *Programmed Proofreading.* Cincinnati, OH, South-Western Publishing Company, 1982.

Preston, Sharon, *Proofreading.* Mountain View, CA, Western Tape, 1977.

## 31—20    REFERENCES FOR THE HANDICAPPED

American Association for Medical Transcription, Visually-Impaired MT Committee, c/o Frances Holland, 635 West Grade, Apt. 306, Chicago, IL 60613.

American Association of Medical Assistants, Inc., *AAMA Guided Study Course: Anatomy, Terminology and Physiology* (cassettes), 20 North Wacker Drive, Chicago, IL 60606.

American Foundation for the Blind, 15 West 16th Street, New York, NY 10011. (annual catalog of publications)

American Printing House for the Blind, P. O. Box 6085, Louisville, KY 40206. (large-print books, books on tape, books put into braille)

Bowe, Frank G., *Personal Computers and Special Needs,* Sybex, Inc., 2021 Challenger Dr., No. 100, Alameda, CA 94501, 1984.

Chabner, Davi-Ellen, Audio tapes to *The Language of Medicine,* W. B. Saunders Company, Independence Square West, Philadelphia, PA 19106-3399.

Clearinghouse-Depository for the Handicapped Student, State Department of Education, 721 Capitol Mall, Sacramento, CA 95814. (for information on large-print books, books on tape, and books put into braille)

Diehl, Marcy O. and Marilyn T. Fordney, *Medical Transcribing Techniques and Procedures,* first ed. on cassettes from Recording for the Blind, Inc., 5022 Hollywood Boulevard, Los Angeles, CA 90027.

Fisher, J. Patrick, *Basic Medical Terminology* (cassettes), The Bobbs-Merrill Educational Publishing Company, 4300 West 62nd Street, Indianapolis, IN 46268.

Gross, Verlee E., *Mastering Medical Terminology* (braille), Braille Institute, 1150 East Fourth Street, Long Beach, CA 90802.

Hollander, Charles S., *Patient's Guide to Vision Rehabilitation for the Partially Sighted,* Sight Improvement Center, Inc., 25 West 43rd Street, New York, NY 10036.

Leonard, Peggy C., *Audio Tapes for Building a Medical Vocabulary,* W. B. Saunders Company, Independence Square West, Philadelphia, PA 19106-3399.

McWilliams, Peter, *Personal Computers and the Disabled,* New York, Doubleday, 1984.

Pyle, Vera, *Current Medical Terminology* (braille), Mrs. Gerri Beeson, Volunteer Services Director, Oklahoma Library for the Blind and Physically Handicapped, 1108 N. E. 36th Street, Oklahoma City, OK 73111.

*Raised Dot Computing Newsletter* (monthly newsletter). 310 South 7th Street, Lewisburg, PA 17837.

Russell, Philip C., *Dynamic Job Interviewing for Women* (braille). Federally Employed Women, P.O. Box 251, Port Hueneme, CA 93041.

Sensory Aids Foundation, 399 Sherman Avenue, Palo Alto, CA 94306. (quarterly journal, research sensory aids, job opportunities, information on latest equipment)

Smith, Genevieve L. and Phyllis E. Davis, *Audio Cassettes for Medical Terminology,* John Wiley and Sons, 330 West State Street, Media, PA 19063.

## 31—21  SELF-EMPLOYMENT AND FREELANCING

Adams, Paul, *The Complete Legal Guide for Your Small Business,* New York, John Wiley and Sons, 1982.

Boos, Patricia, *Typing . . . A Way to Your Own Business,* Bowie, MD, The Seasons Publishing Company, 1981.

DeMenezes, Ruth, *You Can Type for Doctors At Home!,* Thousand Oaks, CA, Claremont Press, 1989.

Murray, Jean Wilson, *Starting and Operating a Word Processing Service,* Babylon, NY, Pilot Books, 1983.

Strickland, Lois, *How to Start a Manuscript Typing Business in Your Home,* 513 Polk Street, Manchester, TN 37355, 1983.

Wisely, Rae, and Gladys Sanders, *The Independent Woman: How to Start and Succeed in Your Own Business,* Los Angeles, Houghton Mifflin Company, 1981.

## 31—22  SPECIALTY REFERENCES

### Dermatology

Leider, Morris, and Morris Rosenblum, *A Dictionary of Dermatological Words, Terms, and Phrases,* West Haven, CT, Dome Laboratories, 1976.

### Gastroenterology

Gastrointestinal Words and Phrases: A Quick Reference Guide; Modesto, CA, Health Professions Institute, 1989.

### History and Physical

Dirckx, John H., M. D., *A Nonphysician's Guide to the Medical History and Physical Examination*, Modesto, CA, Prima Vera Publications, 1987.

### Laboratory

See *Pathology*.

### Obstetrics and Gynecology

Hughes, Edward C., *Obstetric-Gynecologic Terminology with Section on Neonatology and Glossary of Congenital Anomalies*, Philadelphia, F. A. Davis Company, 1972.

### Ophthalmology

Cassin, Barbara, and Sheila Solomon, *Dictionary of Eye Terminology*, Gainesville, FL, Triad Publishing Company, 1984.

DeLorenzo, Barbara and Doris Fedun, *Ophthalmic Terminology*, Thorofare, NJ, Slack, 1988.

Stein, Harold A., Bernard J. Slatt, and Penny Cook, *Manual of Ophthalmic Terminology*, St. Louis, C. V. Mosby Company, 1982.

### Oral and Maxillofacial Surgery

*American Society of Oral Surgeons: The Oral and Maxillofacial Surgery Procedural Terminology with Glossary*, Chicago, American Society of Oral Surgeons, 1975.

## Orthopedics

Blauvelt, Carolyn T., and Fred R. T. Nelson, *A Manual of Orthopaedic Terminology*, St. Louis, C. V. Mosby Company, 1985.

Cittadine, Thomas J., *Orthopedic Terminology*, Thorofare, NJ, Slack, 1988.

Gold Coast Chapter of AAMT, *A Guide to Pathology Terminology*, Fort Lauderdale, FL, Gold Coast Chapter of AAMT, 1984.

Health Professions Institute, *Orthopedic Words and Phrases: A Quick Reference Guide*, Modesto, CA, Health Professions Institute, 1988.

## Pathology

Bennington, James L., *Encyclopedia and Dictionary of Laboratory Medicine and Technology*, Philadelphia, W. B. Saunders Company, 1983.

*Pathology Words and Phrases*, Modesto, CA, Health Professions Institute, 1988.

Sloane, Sheila B. and John L. Dusseau, *A Word Book in Pathology and Laboratory Medicine*, Philadelphia, W. B. Saunders Company, 1984.

Tietz, Norbert W. (ed.), *Clinical Guide to Laboratory Tests*, Philadelphia, W. B. Saunders Company, 1983.

Wallach, Jacques B., *Interpretation of Diagnostic Tests: A Handbook Synopsis of Laboratory Medicine*, Boston, Little, Brown and Company, 1986.

Willatt, E. Murden, *Medical Spelling Handbook, Book 1: Pathology*, Bellaire, TX, Medical Spelling Handbooks Publishing Company, 1970.

## Psychiatry

Hinsie, Leland E., and Robert J. Campbell, *Psychiatric Dictionary*, New York, Oxford University Press, 1970.

Stone, Evelyn M., *American Psychiatric Glossary*, Washington, D.C., American Psychiatric Press, 1988.

## Radiology

Chernok, Norma B., *Radiology Typist's Handbook,* Flushing, NY, Medical Examination Publishing Company, 1970.

Ehlert, Theodora, *Handbook for Medical Secretaries,* Cleveland, Picker Corporation.

Etter, Lewis E., *Glossary of Words and Phrases Used in Radiology, Nuclear Medicine and Ultrasound,* Springfield, IL, Charles C. Thomas, 1970.

Goldman, Myer, and David Cope, *A Radiographic Index,* Littleton, MA, PSG Publishing Company, 1987.

*Radiology Words and Phrases,* Modesto, CA, Health Professional Institute, 1988.

*Roentgenographic Anatomical Terminology,* Wilmington, DE, E.I. DuPont De Nemours and Company.

Sloane, Sheila B., *A Word Book in Radiology With Anatomic Plates and Tables.* Philadelphia, W. B. Saunders Company, 1988.

## Surgery

Chernok, Norma B., *Surgical Typist's Handbook,* Garden City, NY, Medical Examination Publishing Company, 1972.

Coleman, Frances, *Guide to Surgical Terminology,* Oradell, NJ, Medical Economics, 1978.

Smith, E. J. and Y. R. Smith, *Smiths' Reference and Illustrated Guide to Surgical Instruments,* Philadelphia, J. B. Lippincott Company, 1982.

Szulec, Jeanette, and Z. A. Szulec, *Syllabus for the Surgeon's Secretary,* Detroit, The Medical Arts Publishing Company, 1980.

Tessier, Claudia, *The Surgical Word Book,* Philadelphia, W. B. Saunders Company, 1981.

Willatt, E. Murden, *Medical Spelling Handbook, Book 2: Surgery,* Bellaire, TX, Medical Spelling Handbooks Publishing Company, 1970.

## 31—23   SPELLING BOOKS, ENGLISH

Flesch, Rudolf, *Look It Up: A Deskbook of American Spelling and Style,* New York, Harper & Row, 1977.

Gilman, Mary Louise, *One Word, Two Words, Hyphenated?,* National Shorthand Reporters Association, Vienna, Virginia, 1988.

Horowitz, Edward, *Words Come in Families,* New York, A and W Publishers, 1979.

Lewis, Norman, *Correct Spelling Made Easy,* New York, Dell Publishing Company, 1987.

Lewis, Norman, *Instant Spelling Power,* New York, Amsco College Publications, 1976.

## 31—24   SPELLING BOOKS — MEDICAL

American Medical Association, *Current Medical Information and Terminology,* ed. 5, Chicago, American Medical Association, 1981.

Bolander, Donald O. and Rita Bisdorf, *Instant Spelling Medical Dictionary,* Mundelein, IL, Career Publishing Institute, 1970.

Byers, Edward E., *Ten Thousand Medical Words, Spelled and Divided for Quick Reference,* New York, McGraw-Hill Book Company, 1972.

Campbell, Linda C., *The Anatomy Word Book,* Modesto, CA, Prima Vera Publication, 1988.

Carlin, Harriette L., *Medical Secretary Medi-Speller: A Transcription Aid,* Springfield, IL, Charles C. Thomas, 1973.

Cole, Kathleen, and William R. Cole, *Mosby's Medical Speller,* St. Louis, C. V. Mosby Company, 1983.

Coleman, Frances, *Guide to Surgical Terminology,* Oradell, NJ, Medical Economics, 1978.

Cooper, Elsa Swanson, *The Language of Medicine: A Guide for Stenotypists,* Oradell, NJ, Medical Economics, 1977.

*DDC Medical Speller,* Dictation Disc Company, 240 Madison Avenue, New York, NY 10016.

Doyle, John M., and Rita G. Doyle, *Spelling Reference for Business and School,* Reston, VA, Reston Publishing Company, 1976.

Emery, Donald W., *Variant Spellings in Modern American Dictionaries,* Urbana, IL, National Council of Teachers of English, 1973.

Franks, Richard, and H. Swartz, *Simplified Medical Dictionary,* Albany, NY, Medical Economics/Delmar Publishers, 1977. (This book can help you locate a word if you know how the word ends and how the beginning is pronounced. The terms are categorized by their prefixes, suffixes, and roots, so you can seek out the word with minimal effort.)

*Glossary of Hospital Terms,* Chicago, IL, American Medical Record Association, 1974.

Hafer, Ann, *The Medical and Health Sciences Word Book,* Boston, Houghton Mifflin Company, 1982.

Johnson, Carrie E., *Medical Spelling Guide,* Springfield, IL, Charles C. Thomas, 1966.

Kreivsky, Joseph, and Jordon L. Linfield, *The Bad Speller's Dictionary,* New York, Random House, 1974.

Lee, Richard V. and Doris J. Hofer, *How to Divide Medical Words,* Carbondale, IL, Southern Illinois University Press, 1972.

Lorenzini, Jean W., *Medical Phrase Index,* Oradell, NJ, Medical Economics, 1989.

Magalini, Sergio I. and Euclide Scrascia, *Dictionary of Medical Syndromes,* Philadelphia, J. B. Lippincott Company, 1981.

Mullins, Nancy L. (ed.), *Mosby's Medical Speller,* St. Louis, C. V. Mosby Company, 1983.

Pease, Roger W., Jr. (ed.), *Webster's Medical Speller,* Springfield, IL, G & C Merriam Company, 1975.

Prichard, Robert W. and Robert E. Robinson, *Twenty Thousand Medical Words,* New York, McGraw-Hill Book Company, 1972.

Pyle, Vera, *Current Medical Terminology,* Modesto, CA, Prima Vera Publications, 1988.

Rimer, Evelyn Harbeck, *Harbeck's Glossary of Medical Terms,* Brisbane, CA, San Francisco WEB Offset, 1967.

Sloane, Sheila B., *The Medical Word Book,* ed. 2., Philadelphia, W. B. Saunders Company, 1982.

Tessier, Claudia J., *The Surgical Word Book,* Philadelphia, W. B. Saunders Company, 1981.

Willeford, George Jr., *Webster's New World Medical Word Finder,* Englewood Cliffs, NJ, Prentice-Hall, 1987.

Willey, Joy, *Glossary of Medical Terminology for the Health Professions,* Thorofare, NJ, Slack, 1988.

## 31—25 STYLE MANUALS — MEDICAL AND GENERAL

American Medical Association, *Style Book/Editorial Manual of the American Medical Association,* Littleton, MA, Publishing Sciences Group, 1976.

*American Psychological Association: Publication Manual,* Washington, D.C., American Psychological Association, 1974.

Barclay, William R., et al., compiled for American Medical Association, *Manual for Authors and Editors: Editorial Style and Manuscript Preparation,* Los Altos, CA, Lange Medical Publications, 1981.

*The Chicago Manual of Style,* Chicago, University of Chicago Press, 1982.

*Council of Biology Editors Committee on Form and Style: CBE Style Manual,* Washington, D.C., American Institute of Biological Sciences, 1974.

Ebbitt, Wilma R. and David Ebbitt, *Writer's Guide and Index to English,* Glenview, IL, Scott, Foresman and Company, 1982.

Huth, Edward J., M. D., *Medical Style and Format — An International Manual for Authors, Editors, and Publishers,* Philadelphia, Institute for Scientific Information Press, 1987.

Preston, Sharon. *Proofreading,* Mountain View, CA, Western Tape, 1977.

Schramm, Dwane, *Typing Term Papers and Reports,* Mountain View, CA, Western Tape, 1974.

Strunk, William, Jr., and E. B. White, *The Elements of Style: With Index,* New York, Macmillan Publishing Company, 1979.

Tessier, Claudia, and Sally C. Pitman, *Style Guide for Medical Transcription,* Modesto, CA, American Association for Medical Transcription, 1985.

Trelease, S. F., *How to Write Scientific and Technical Papers,* Cambridge, MA, MIT Press, 1969.

*Webster's Standard American Style Manual,* Springfield, MA, Merriam-Webster, 1985.

## 31—26 TYPING AND TRANSCRIPTION

Diehl, Marcy O. and Marilyn T. Fordney, *Medical Typing and Transcribing Techniques and Procedures,* Philadelphia, W. B. Saunders Company, 1984.

## 31—27    WORD DIVISION

Byers, Edward E., *Ten Thousand Medical Words, Spelled and Divided for Quick Reference*, New York, McGraw-Hill Book Company, 1972.

Hafer, Ann, *The Medical and Health Sciences Word Book*, Boston, Houghton Mifflin Company, 1982.

Lee, Richard B. and Doris J. Hofer, *How to Divide Medical Words*, Carbondale, IL, Southern Illinois University Press, 1972.

Pease, Roger W., Jr. (ed.), *Webster's Medical Speller*, Springfield, MA, G & C Merriam Company, 1975.

Silverthorn, J. E. and Devern J. Perry, *Word Division Manual*, Cincinnati, South-Western Publishing Company, 1970.

Willeford, George, Jr., *Webster's New World Medical Word Finder*, Englewood Cliffs, NJ, Prentice-Hall, 1987.

*The Word Book II*, Boston, Houghton Mifflin Company, 1983.

Zoubek, C. E. and G. A. Condon, *Twenty Thousand Words*, New York, McGraw-Hill Book Company, 1985.

## 31—28    WRITING — SCIENTIFIC AND TECHNICAL

Alvarez, Joseph A., *Elements of Technical Writing*, Albany, NY, Academic Press, 1986.

Brogan, John A., *Clear Technical Writing*, New York, McGraw-Hill Book Company, 1973.

Dagher, Joseph P., *Technical Communication: A Practical Guide*, Englewood Cliffs, NJ, Prentice-Hall, 1978.

Ehrlich, Eugene H. and Daniel Murphy, *Art of Technical Writing: A Manual for Scientists, Engineers, and Students*, Scranton, PA, Apollo Editions, 1969.

King, Lester S., *Why Not Say It Clearly: A Guide to Scientific Writing*, Boston, Little, Brown and Company, 1978.

Mitchell, John H., *Writing for Technical and Professional Journals*, Ann Arbor, MI, Books Demand UMI, 1968.

Skillin, Marjorie, and Robert Gay, *Words Into Type*, Englewood Cliffs, NJ, Prentice Hall, 1974.

Trelease, Sam F., *How to Write Scientific and Technical Papers*, Cambridge, MA, MIT Press, 1969.

# 32

# Semicolon

## 32—1   INDEPENDENT CLAUSE WITH NO CONJUNCTION

**DO**   use a semicolon to separate two or more closely related independent clauses when there is no conjunction used.

You have requested our cooperation; we have complied.

The nose is remarkable for loud congestive breathing; there is no discharge visible.

**NOTE.**   *Usually, you can also use a period and make two sentences.*

The nose is remarkable for loud congestive breathing. There is no discharge visible.

**OPTION.**   *use a comma to separate two independent clauses when the sentences are very brief and closely related.*

She was in today for follow-up exam, she was doing well.

# 32 SEMICOLON

## 32—2  INDEPENDENT CLAUSE HEAVILY PUNCTUATED

**_DO_**    use a semicolon to separate independent clauses if either one or both of them have been punctuated with two or more commas.

Around the first of July, he developed pain in his chest, which he ignored for several days; and, finally, he saw me, at the request of his family doctor, on July 16.

## 32—3  SERIES WITH PUNCTUATION

**_DO_**    use a semicolon between a series of phrases or clauses if any item in the series has internal commas.

Among those present at the Utilization Committee Meeting were Dr. Frank Byron, chief-of-staff; Mrs. Joan Armath, administrator; Ms. Nancy Speeth, medical records technician; and Mr. Ralph Johnson, director of nurses.

## 32—4  WITH TRANSITIONAL EXPRESSIONS

**_DO_**    use a semicolon **before** a transitional expression when it is used to join two independent clauses.

**DO**    use a comma **after** the expression when it is composed of two or more syllables.

I attempted a labor induction with Pitocin, and contractions occurred; however, the patient failed to develop an effective labor pattern, and I discharged her after eight hours.

*NOTE.* *Some of the most common conjunctive adverbs used as transitional expressions are* however, furthermore, nevertheless, therefore, consequently, accordingly, anyhow, still, *and* then.

## 32—5    WITH QUOTATION MARKS AND PARENTHESES

**DO**    place the semicolon outside quotation marks and parentheses.

# 33

# Slang

# and

# Unusual

# Medical

# Terms

## INTRODUCTION

Sometimes a physician will dictate an unusual expression that may puzzle you and you may try to find it in a medical or English reference book. Chances are you will not find the expression and will type the phrase the way you heard it and/or flag it for the physician to double check. See also Chapter 10, *Editing*.

**_DO_**  check with your supervisor before transcribing or editing questionable slang.

The patient was stupid, a crock (hypochondriac), and dumb.

**_DO_**   contact the dictator and diplomatically and tactfully question his or her use of the slang expression before it becomes a permanent part of the patient's medical record.

## 33—1   ACRONYMS

**_DO_**   spell out or abbreviate medical acronyms in medical reports.

The patient was given a CABG. (correct)
The patient was given a coronary artery bypass graft. (correct)

## 33—2   BRIEF FORMS

**_DO_**   translate slang terms in full when dictated.

Appy should be typed as appendectomy.
Cathed should be typed as catheterized.
Dex should be typed as dexamethasone.
H. flu should be typed as *H. influenzae* or
    *Hemophilus influenzae.*
Lab may be typed as laboratory.
Lytes should be typed as electrolytes.

**_DO_**   edit slang words and phrases.

She failed to hand me the Mets (or Metz) scissors. (incorrect)
She failed to hand me the Metzenbaum scissors. (correct)

Mrs. Becker's temp was 102°. (incorrect)
Mrs. Becker's temperature was 102°. (correct)

At the end of surgery, I introduced an intracath. (incorrect)
At the end of surgery, I introduced an intravenous catheter. (correct)

## 33—3   FLAGGING, CARDING, TAGGING, OR MARKING

**_DO_**     flag, tag, or mark a slang expression if you cannot
translate the slang term in full, and leave a blank. Attach a note to the transcript with a brief description of
where the blank is located.

See Figure 10–1.

## 33—4   PUNCTUATION

**_DO_**     use quotation marks to enclose slang, coined,
awkward, whimsical, or humorous words that might
show ignorance on the part of the writer if it is not
known that he/she is aware of them.

See if you can schedule a few "well" patients for a
change.

If you have "clergyman's knee," "tailor's seat," "tennis elbow," or "trigger finger," what you really have is
a form of bursitis or tendinitis.

## 33—5   SLANG TERMS

Some of the unusual terms commonly dictated in medical
reports are listed in Table 33–1 to help you through puzzling dictation. To give you a clue as to when these slang expressions
might be used, the type of specialist or a brief definition of the
term is given in the right hand column. These dictated words and
phrases are usually typed as shown. Remember, it is optional to
abbreviate or spell out acronyms.

# 33 SLANG AND UNUSUAL MEDICAL TERMS

Table 33–1. Unusual Terms Commonly Dictated in Medical Reports

| Term | Specialist/Definition |
| --- | --- |
| acorn tipped catheter | urologist |
| Ambu bag | (a low-tech resuscitation tool in the emergency room) |
| angle of Louis | surgeon |
| argyle tube | surgeon |
| ash leaf spots (eye) | ophthalmologist |
| BABYbird respirator | respiratory system |
| banana blade knife | orthopedist |
| banjo-string adhesions | surgeon |
| basement membrane | nephrologist, ophthalmologist |
| Best clamps | surgeon |
| bikini bottom | orthopedist |
| Billroth II (procedure) | gastroenterologist/surgeon |
| Bird machine (on the Bird) | respiratory system |
| black doggie clamps | clamps |
| black heel | orthopedist |
| blowout fracture | orthopedist |
| blue bloaters | radiologist |
| bony thorax | orthopedist |
| brawny edema or brawny induration | skin (a general term) |
| bucket-handle tear | orthopedist |
| buffy coat | pathologist |
| CABG (pronounced "cabbage") refers to coronary artery bypass graft | cardiologist |
| CAT scan | radiologist |
| chain cystogram | urologist |
| charley horse | orthopedist |
| choked disc (or disk) | ophthalmologist |
| cigarette (or cigaret) drain | surgeon |
| clap (gonorrhea) | gynecologist/urologist |
| clergyman's knee | orthopedist |
| clog (clot of blood) | cardiovascular surgeon |
| coffee-ground stools | gastroenterologist |
| cogwheel rigidity or motion | hemologist |
| cottonoid patty | surgeon |
| COWS | refers to cold to the opposite, warm to the same — a mnemonic device used in otolaryngology for the Hallpike caloric stimulation response |
| crick (painful spasm in a muscle, usually in the neck) | orthopedist |

| Term | Specialist/Definition |
|------|----------------------|
| Dandy scissors | surgeon |
| doll's eye movements | neurologist |
| fat pad | orthopedist |
| fat towels (wound towels) | surgeon |
| fern test (an estrogen test) | gynecologist |
| finger clubbing | pediatrician, orthopedist |
| fish-mouthed cervix | obstetrician/gynecologist |
| flashers and floaters (eye exam) | ophthalmologist |
| 49er brace | orthopedist |
| frank breech position | obstetrician |
| gallops, thrills, and rubs | respiratory system |
| gimpy (lame) | orthopedist |
| glitter cells | pathologist |
| goose egg (swelling due to blunt trauma) | orthopedist |
| gull-wing sign | neurologist |
| guy suture | surgeon |
| haircut (syphilitic chancre) | — |
| hammock configuration | — |
| hanging drop test | pathologist |
| hickey | dermatologist |
| His (bundle) | cardiologist |
| hot potato voice | otolaryngologist |
| jogger's nipples | orthopedist |
| joint mice | orthopedist |
| Kerley's B lines (costophrenic septal lines) | radiologist |
| Kerley's C lines | radiologist |
| kick counts | obstetrician |
| lacer cock-up (splint) | orthopedist |
| lemon squeezer (instrument) | vascular surgeon |
| Little lens | ophthalmologist |
| loose body | orthopedist |
| Mill-house murmur | cardiologist |
| mouse (periorbital ecchymosis) | ophthalmologist |
| mouse units | laboratory |
| MUGA | cardiologist |
| Mule vitreous sphere | ophthalmologist |
| musical bruit | cardiologist |
| Mustard procedure | vascular surgeon |
| octopus test | ophthalmologist |
| outrigger (orthopedic) | orthopedist |
| ox cell hemolysin test | pathologist |

*Table continues on next page*

**Table 33–1.** *Continued*

| Term | Specialist/Definition |
| --- | --- |
| oyster (mass of mucus coughed up) | respiratory system |
| pants-over-vest (technique) | surgeon |
| parrot beak tear | orthopedist |
| patient flat lined ("expired" is preferred) | a general term |
| peanut (a small surgical gauze sponge) | surgeon |
| peanut forceps (instrument) | surgeon |
| PERLA or PERRLA | (pupils equal, regular, react to light and to accommodation) |
| piggyback prove | |
| pigtail catheter | cardiovascular surgeon |
| piles (hemorrhoids) | proctologist |
| pill-rolling (tremor) | neurologist |
| pink puffer (patient showing dyspnea but no cyanosis) | cardiologist |
| pins and needles (paresthesias) | neurologist |
| pollywogs (cotton pledgets or sponges with pointed ends) | surgeon |
| prep or prepped (from the word "prepared") | surgeon |
| prostate boggy | urologist |
| proudflesh (granulation tissue) | surgeon |
| prune belly syndrome | endocrinologist |
| pulmonary toilet | pulmonologist |
| purse-string suture | surgeon |
| rocker-bottom foot | orthopedist |
| romied from an acronym: R = rule, O = out, M = myocardial, | cardiologist |
| I = infarction | cardiologist |
| rooting reflex | pediatrician |
| rubber booties | surgeon |
| rugger jersey sign | — |
| runner's rump | orthopedist |
| running off (diarrhea) | gastroenterologist |
| salmon flesh excrescences | — |
| sand (encrusted secretions about the eyes) | ophthalmologist |
| saucerize | refers to suturing a cyst inside out so it will heal |

| Term | Specialist/Definition |
|------|----------------------|
| scotty dog's ear | surgeon |
| seagull bruit | respiratory system, cardiologist |
| shiner | black eye or hematoma of eye |
| shoelace suturing | surgeon |
| shotty nodes or shoddy nodes | a general term |
| simian crease (seen in Down syndrome) | pediatrician |
| skin wheals | dermatologist |
| skinny needle or Chiba needle | surgeon |
| sky suture | surgeon |
| sleep (inspissated mucus about the eyes) | a general term |
| smile or smiling incision | surgeon |
| smoker's face | a general term |
| snowball opacities | ophthalmologist |
| snowbanks | ophthalmologist |
| snuff box | orthopedist |
| steeple sign (on chest x-ray) | radiologist |
| stick-tie | refers to suture ligature, transfixion suture, or a long strand of suture clamped on a hemostat) |
| stonebasket | urologist |
| stoved (of a finger) means stubbed | orthopedist |
| string sign | radiologist |
| sugar-tong plaster splint | orthopedist |
| sugar tongs (instrument) | orthopedist |
| "surf" test (surfactant test of amniotic fluid) | pathologist |
| tailor's seat | orthopedist |
| tennis elbow | orthopedist |
| trick (of a joint) means unstable | orthopedist |
| trigger finger | orthopedist |
| tumor plot | cardiologist |
| two-flight dyspnea | respiratory system |
| two-pillow orthopnea | respiratory system |
| walking pneumonia | respiratory system |
| weaver's bottom | orthopedist |
| wet mount | pathologist |
| wing suture | surgeon |
| witches milk | neonatologist |
| yoga foot drop | orthopedist |
| ZEEP (zero end respiratory pressure) | pulmonologist |
| zit (comedo) | dermatologist |

# 34

## $S_{LASH}$

## INTRODUCTION

The slash is also called the diagonal, bar, virgule, slant, or solidus. The slash is typed with no space on either side.

## 34—1   FRACTIONS

**_DO_**     use the slash to write fractions.

2/3    1 1/2

**DON'T**   mix keyboard fractions and those made by typing each number.

They measured out at ¼, 1/3, ½. (incorrect)

They measured out at $\frac{1}{4}$  $\frac{1}{3}$  $\frac{1}{2}$ . (incorrect)

They measured out at 1/4, 1/3, 1/2. (correct)

## 34—2   SEPARATING CERTAIN TECHNICAL TERMS

**_DO_**   use the slash in writing certain technical terms. The slash sometimes substitutes for the words *per*, to, or *over*.

She has 20/20 vision. (separates the indicators of visual acuity)

His blood pressure is 120/80. (takes the place of the word *over*)

Grade II/IV systolic murmur (takes the place of the word *over*)

The dosage is 50 mg/day. (takes the place of the word *per*)

Please note the A/B ratio. (takes the place of the word *to*)

**DON'T**   use the slash to take the place of *per* except in describing **specific** quantities and a **form of measurement** (including time) which can then be correctly used in an abbreviated form immediately preceding the slash.

He has been smoking three packs of cigarettes per day. (correct)

He has been smoking three packs of cigarettes/day. (incorrect)

Turn it a centimeter per day.

*or*

Turn it 1 cm/day. (correct)

*NOTE.* *Avoid using the slash to separate parts of a date when typing chart notes. Dates should be spelled out in medical reports, memos, and letters.*

4/6/94 (may cause some misinterpretation with the slash being read as the number one [1])

4-6-94 (better and acceptable for chart notes)

April 6, 1994 (first choice in text material)

**DON'T**     use the slash to express a ratio (see Rule 5–5).

serum was diluted 1/200,000 (incorrect)
serum was diluted 1:200,000 (correct)

a 1/2 dilute solution was used (incorrect)
a 1:2 dilute solution was used (correct)

***DO***     use the slash in making the abbreviation for the expression *in care of* in an address.

Ms. Margot Hunter
c/o J. B. Marsh
2387 First Street
La Mesa, CA 92041

### 34—3     WORD CHOICE

***DO***     use the slash to offer word choice.

and/or
he/she
his/her
Mr./Mrs./Miss/Ms.
+/−
plus/minus

# 35

## $S$PACING

## WITH

## PUNCTUATION

## MARKS

## 35—1    NO SPACE

following a period within an abbreviation
following a period used as a decimal point
between quotation marks and the quoted material
before or after a hyphen
before or after a slash
before or after a dash (two hyphens)
between parentheses and the enclosed material
between any word and the punctuation following it
between the number and the colon in a dilute
solution
on either side of the colon when expressing the time
of day

# 35

## 35—2    ONE SPACE

after a comma
after a semicolon
after a period following an initial
after the closing parenthesis

## 35—3    TWO SPACES

after a period, question mark, or exclamation point at the end of a sentence.

after a quotation mark at the end of a sentence

after a colon (except when used with the time of day or when expressing a dilute solution)

# 36

# Spelling

## INTRODUCTION

**_DO_**  verify the spelling of a word in an English or medical dictionary when in doubt about its spelling.

# 36 SPELLING

**DON'T** accept the spelling of a word given by the dictator or anyone else unless you know it is correct or have checked it in a reference source.

**_DO_** use the medical spelling of a word when there is a difference between spellings given by the medical dictionary and the English dictionary.

## 36—1 ANATOMIC WORDS

**_DO_** type out English and Latin names of anatomic parts as dictated.

abductor hallucis muscle        basalis vein
femoralis nerve                 infraorbitalis artery

## 36—2 BRITISH WORDS

When submitting a manuscript to a British journal, these rules may come in handy for reference, since words in the manuscript must conform to British rules. In addition, all names of drugs mentioned in the manuscript must also be listed according to the drug name as known in Great Britain.

**_DO_** spell the suffix -*ize* as -*ise* when pronounced "eyes."

rationalize, rationalization (American spelling)
rationalise, rationalisation (British spelling)

**_DO_** use the preferred spelling for the suffix -*lyze* as -*lyse*.

analyze (American preference)
analyse (British preference)

**DO** include an internal *-e* when words are derived from stems ending in a silent *-e* by adding *-able* or *-ment*.

likable (American spelling)
likeable (British spelling)

judgment (American preference)
judgement (British spelling)

*EXCEPTION.*   *Lovable (British spelling)*

**DO** watch doubling or nondoubling of consonants.

fulfill (American spelling)
fulfil (British spelling)

skillful (American spelling
skilful (British spelling)

**DO** watch variances in spelling that differ in phonetic sounds.

jail (American spelling)   gaol (British spelling)

curb (American spelling)   kerb (British spelling)

mold (American spelling)   mould (British spelling)

**DO** use British digraphs *ae* and *oe* for medical terms.

anesthesia (American spelling)   anaesthesia (British spelling)

orthopedic (American spelling)   orthopaedic (British spelling) hematology (American spelling) haematology (British spelling)

esophagus (American spelling)   oesophagus (British spelling)

rectocele (American spelling) rectocoele (British spelling)

**_DO_**     spell some British technical words without digraph elements differently than the American spelling.

aluminum (American spelling)   aluminium (British spelling)

**_DO_**     spell titles and proper names when mentioned in text, tables, or cited in references by retaining their original spelling.

*Haemophilus influenzae* (American and British spelling)

**_DO_**     consult *Butterworth's Medical Dictionary, Chambers 20th Century Dictionary,* or *International Dictionary of Medicine and Biology* for British spelling.

## 36—3   COMPOUND WORDS

See Chapter 7, *Compounds.*

## 36—4   CONSONANTS

**_DO_**   double the final consonant of a one-syllable word before adding a suffix beginning with a vowel if the final consonant is preceded by a single vowel.

redd-er        plott- ed        cutt-ing        gass-ed

**EXCEPTION.**  *Before the plural ending -es, the final consonant remains single.*

bus-es        gas-es

**DON'T**   double the final consonant if the final consonant is preceded by another consonant or by two vowels.

loo k        loo ked

**_DO_**   double the final consonant of a word of more than one syllable before adding a suffix beginning with a vowel if the final consonant is preceded by a vowel and the word is accented on the last syllable.

| | | | |
|---|---|---|---|
| control' | controlling | controlled | |
| curet' | curet*ting* | curetted | curettage |
| refer' | referring | referred | |

**EXCEPTION.**  *Reference.*

**_DO_**   double the final l before a suffix even when the root word is not accented on the last syllable.

gravell-y        tonsillitis

# 36 SPELLING

**DON'T** double the final consonant when the accent does not fall on the last syllable or the final consonant is preceded by another consonant.

tra' vel        trave ler

**DON'T** double a consonant after a long vowel.

apical          celiac          contusion          pilonidal

**_EXCEPTIONS._** _Bass, gross, dissect._

**DON'T** double the final consonant before any suffix when a word of one or more syllables ends with more than one consonant.

back            back _ward_
return          return _ed_
mass            mass _ive_

**_NOTE._** _Words that end in_ ll _generally keep both consonants before a suffix. However, when adding the suffix_ -ly _drop one_ l _from the root word. When adding the suffixes_ -less _or_ -like, _insert a hypen to avoid three_ l's _in a row._

chill           chilly          cell            cell-like
full            fully           cooly

## 36—5    DIACRITICAL MARKS

**_DO_** add an _e_ if your word processor or computer software cannot place an umlaut ( ¨ ) over _a, o,_ or _u._

Pötzsch         Poetzsch

**DON'T**  add an accent mark to most English words taken from French, Spanish, or other foreign languages.

Type: apropos, boutonniere, cabana, cafe, coupe, facade, matinee, melee, puree, role, smorgasbord, soiree, vicuna.

***DO***  type these foreign words with their accents (´) (`) (~).

à la carte, à la mode, attaché, cause célèbre, chargé d'affaires, mañana, outré, passé, pâté, père, piéce de résistance, pied-à -terre, touché, vis-à -vis.

***DO***  type these French phrases with a circumflex ( ^ ).

bête noire, maître d'hôtel, pâté, raison d'être, table d'hôte, tête-à -tête.

## 36—6  DRUG NAMES

See Chapter 9, *Drugs and Drug References.*

## 36—7  EI AND IE WORDS

***DO***  use *i* before *e* except after *c* or when sounded like *a,* as in *neighbor* and *weigh.*

| | | | | |
|---|---|---|---|---|
| ie: chief | believe | relief | hygiene | |
| ei: receive | conceive | weigh | neighbor | vein |

**EXCEPTIONS.**  *Financier, either, leisure, neither, seize, weird.*

**DO**       spell most words *ei* that have long *i* syllables.

      height

**DO**       spell most words *ei* that have long *e* syllables.

      caffeine     codeine     protein

**DO**       use *ie* after the letter *c* when *c* is pronounced like "sh."

      efficient     deficient

## 36—8     EPONYMS

See Chapter 12, *Eponyms.*

## 36—9     FINAL SILENT *e*

**DO**       keep the *e* before a suffix beginning with a consonant, but drop the *e* before a suffix beginning with a vowel (*-ing, -able, -er, -ed, -or*, and so forth) for words ending in silent *e*.

| improve | improve *ment* | |
|---------|----------------|----------|
| operate | opera *tion* | operat *or* |
| pale | pale *ness* | |
| use | us *able* | us *ing* |

**EXCEPTIONS.** *After* c *or* g, *if the suffix begins with* a *or* o, *the* e *is kept.*

notice     noticeable

*Keep the* e *when dropping it causes confusion with another word.*

dye     dyeing     (Not: dying)

*If the word ends in* oe, *the* e *is kept.*

hoe     hoeing     (Not: hoeed or hooer)

## 36—10     FRENCH MEDICAL WORDS

***DO***

take special care in spelling French medical words because different sounds are given to the letters. See also Rule 36–5.

ballottement (pronounced bah-LOT-maw or bah-LOT-ment)
bougie (pronounced boo-ZHE, BOO-zhe, or BOO-je)
bougienage (pronounced boo-zhe-NAHZH)
bruit (pronounced brwe or broot)
cafe-au-lait (pronounced kah-FAY-o-LAY)
chancre (pronounced SHANG-ker)
contrecoup or contracoup (pronounced kon-tr-KOO)
cul-de-sac (pronounced KUL-de-sahk)
curette or curet (pronounced ku-RET)
debridement (pronounced da-BRED-maw or de-BRIDE-ment)
douche (pronounced doosh)
gastrogavage (pronounced gas"tro-gah-VAHZH)
gastrolavage (pronounced gas"tro-lah-VAHZH)
lavage (pronounced lah-VAHZH or LAV-ij)
milieu (pronounced me-LOO)
peau d'orange (pronounced po-do-RAHNJ)
poudrage (pronounced poo-DRAHZH)
rale (pronounced rahl)
Roux-en-Y (pronounced ROO-en-why)
tic douloureux (pronounded tik doo-loo-ROO)
triage (pronounced tre-AHZH)

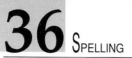 

## 36—11 HOMONYMS

See also *Common Medical Homonyms* (appendix). For a reference book, see Rule 31–3.

**_DO_**    look up the meaning of English and medical homonyms to end confusion and help you decide how to spell them. Homonyms sound the same but have different meanings.

## 36—12 NOUNS TO VERBS

**_DO_**    use an English rule to spell a verb that the dictator has created from a noun or trade name.

| | |
|---|---|
| pedicle (noun) | pedicleized (verb) |
| Hyfrecator (trade name) | hyfrecated (verb) |
| Bovie (trade name) | bovied (verb) |
| saucer (noun) | saucerize (verb) |

*NOTE. Some physicians have coined verbs from acronyms. These should usually be spelled out in full regardless of the dictation.*

*EXCEPTION. When the physician dictates PERRLA (pupils equal, regular, react to light and to accommodation) when doing a physical examination on a patient, the acronym PERRLA may be typed into the report.*

The patient was admitted with severe precordial pain and cardiac arrhythmias and was romied. (R = rule, O = out, M = myocardial, I = infarction).

The patient was CABG'd. (C = coronary, A = artery, B = bypass, G = graft).

Blood had proetzed into the sinus cavity. (from Proetz method of injecting fluid by pressure into a cavity)

## 36—13   ONE WORD, TWO WORDS, OR HYPHENATED

See also Chapter 15, *Hyphen Use and Word Division* or obtain one of the following books: *Look It Up: A Deskbook of American Spelling and Style* by Rudolf Flesch, Harper and Row, Publishers, New York, New York, 1977; *One Word, Two Words, Hyphenated?* by Mary Louise Gilman, National Shorthand Reporters Association, Vienna, Virginia, 1988.

The following is a list of medical words commonly encountered that typists have trouble in remembering whether to type as two words, a hyphenated word, or one word.

afterload
bed rest (1 or 2 words,
    depends on reference used)
bedsores
breakdown (noun)
breastbone
breast-feeding
checkup
cheekbone
chickenpox
chin bone
clear-cut
cogwheel
dipstick
downgoing
eardrum
earwax
face lift (1 or 2 words,
    depends on reference used)
fiber optic (1 or 2 words,
    depends on reference used)
fingernail
fingertip
follow-up (adjective);
    followup (noun);
    follow up (verb)
footdrop

gallbladder
headrest
herpesvirus
inpatient
lid lag
lightheaded
middorsal
nail plate
nonmedical
nose drops
outpatient
pacemaker
piggyback
pigskin (adjective)
pigtail (adjective)
postoperative
preoperative
pursestring (noun); purse-string
    (adjective)
reexamine
sea fronds
seagull bruit
take down of fistula (1 or 2
    words, depends on
    reference used)
water-hammer (adjective)
zigzag incision

## 36—14    PLURALS

See Chapter 25, *Plural Forms*

## 36—15    PREFIXES

**_DO_**    retain the consonant or vowel when attaching a prefix that brings identical letters into contact.

dissociation    reexcitation    salpingo-oophorectomy

**NOTE.**   *Doubling of an initial consonant does not occur as a result of adding a prefix except with Greek initial* rh.

rhythm      arrhythmia

**EXCEPTION.**   *Biorhythm*

**_DO_**    change the *d* in the prefix *ad-* to a *c, f, g, p, s,* or *t* before words beginning with those consonants.

afferent          accident        agglutination
appointment       assist          attend

**_DO_**    change the *con-* to *co-* before vowels or *h* to *col-* before *l*; to *com-* before *b, m,* or *p*; and to *cor-* before *r*.

contraction   coalesce   coaptation   coarctation
corrugation  commissurotomy  collateral  connective

**_DO_**    delete the *n* in the prefix *syn-* when it appears before *s*, change it to *l* before *l*, and change it to *m* before *b, m, p,* and *ph*.

systaltic   symphysis   symblepharon   symmetry

**_DO_**   change the *n* in the prefix *en-* to an *m* before *b*, *p*, or *ph*.

engorgement    emphlysis

**_DO_**   change the *n* in the prefix *in-* to an *m* before *b*, *p*, or *m*; change the *n* to an *l* or *r* before words beginning with those consonants.

infiltration    insertion    irradiation    immersion

**_DO_**   change the *b* in the prefix *ob-* to a *c* before words beginning with that consonant.

obtuse    occlude

## 36—16   REFERENCES FOR SPELLING WORDS

See Chapter 31, *Reference Materials and Publications.*

## 36—17   SILENT CONSONANTS

**_DO_**   use Chapter 41, *Word Finder*, to learn spelling possibilities for silent consonants so that a word can be located in the medical dictionary. Examples of words with silent consonants follow:

| Spelling at Beginning of Word | Phonetic Sound | Example |
|---|---|---|
| pn | n | pneumonia |
| ps | s | psychiatric |
| pt | t | ptosis |
| ct | t | ctetology |
| cn | n | cnemis |
| gn | n | gnathalgia |
| mn | n | mnemonic |
| kn | n | knuckle |

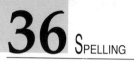

## 36—18    SLANG AND UNUSUAL MEDICAL TERMS

See Chapter 33, *Slang and Unusual Medical Terms.*

## 36—19    WORDS ENDING IN -ABLE AND -IBLE

**_DO_**    end words in -able when the root is a complete word.

adapt    adaptable

**_DO_**    end words in *-able* when the *final e* has been dropped and the root is a complete word.

advise    advisable

**_DO_**    change the last letter in root words that end in *i or y* to an *i* and add -able.

rely        reliable
deny        deniable

**_DO_**    end words in *-able* when the root ends in *hard c* (as in *cough*) or *hard g* (as in *big*).

practicable    navigable

*NOTE.* *Exceptions to the preceding rules follow:*

| | | | |
|---|---|---|---|
| affable | equitable | inflammable | memorable |
| amenable | exchangeable | inscrutable | palpable |
| capable | formidable | inseparable | peaceable |
| changeable | hospitable | intolerable | portable |
| chargeable | indomitable | malleable | probable |
| controllable | inevitable | manageable | unpronounceable |
| enforceable | inexorable | marriageable | vulnerable |

**DO**  end a word in *-ible* when the root is *not a complete* word.

    audible       edible       possible

**DO**  end a word in *-ible* when the root is a complete word that has *-ive* or *-ion* in one of its forms.

    digest       digestive       digestion       digestible

*EXCEPTIONS.* *Correctable, predictable.*

**DO**  end a word in *-ible* when the root ends in *-ns* or *-ss.*

    insensible       admissible

*EXCEPTION.* *Indispens*able, *which is related to dispensation. If any form of the word has a long* a, *the word takes the* -able *ending.*

**DO**  end a word in *-ible* when the root ends in *soft c* (as in *reduce*) or *soft g* (as in *ginger*).

    forcible       negligible

*NOTE.* *Exceptions to the preceding rules follow:*

| | |
|---|---|
| collaps *ible* | flex *ible* |
| contempt *ible* | gull *ible* |
| convert *ible* | inflex *ible* |
| divis *ible* | irresist *ible* |
| discern *ible* | revers *ible* |

*NOTE.* *-ible words are rarer than -able words.*

---

## 36—20    WORDS ENDING IN -ANT/-ANCE and -ENT/-ENCE

**_DO_**    use *-ant*, *-ance*, or *-ancy* when the suffix is preceded by *c* having the sound of *k*, or *g* having a hard sound.

significant    vacancy

**_DO_**    use *-ent*, *-ence*, or *-ency* when *c* has the sound of *s*, or *g* the sound of *j*.

convalescent    negligence    indigent

**_DO_**    consult the dictionary if the suffix is preceded by a letter other than *c* or *g* and you are in doubt about the spelling as there are no clear-cut rules.

---

## 36—21    WORDS ENDING IN -CEDE, -CEED, AND -SEDE

**_DO_**    use the suffix *-sede* on the word *supersede*, as it is the only word in the English language spelled with that suffix.

**_DO_**  use the suffix -ceed with only these three words: ex-ceed, proceed, and succeed. Do spell all others with -cede (precede, recede, and so forth).

## 36—22  WORDS ENDING IN -C

**_DO_**  add the letter _k_ before a suffix with words ending in _c_.

| | | |
|---|---|---|
| panic | panicked | panicking   panicky |
| mimic | mimicked | mimicking (Exception: mimicry) |

*EXCEPTION.*  *Arc, arced, arcing.*

## 36—23  WORDS ENDING IN -D OR -T

**_DO_**  change the _d_ or _t_ of a root to _s_ before the suffix -ion.

| | |
|---|---|
| corrod | corroSION |
| erod | eroSION |
| convert | converSION |
| pervert | perverSION |

*NOTE.*  *Exceptions to the preceding rule follow:*

| | |
|---|---|
| digest | digestion |
| perfect | perfection |
| corrupt | corruption |
| destruct | destruction |

*NOTE.*  *The "shun" sound may be spelled in a variety of ways. Unless you are certain of the correct spelling of this ending, consult your dictionary.*

permission  dietitian  flexion  complexion

---

## 36—24    WORDS ENDING IN -EFY AND -IFY

---

**_DO_**    use *-efy* to spell the four words (*liquefy, putrefy, rarefy,* and *stupefy*) that end in the suffix *-efy*. All other words in this category end in *-ify* (*clarify, testify,* and so forth).

---

## 36—25    WORDS ENDING IN -Y

---

**_DO_**    change the *y* to an *i* before adding a suffix except when a suffix beginning with *i* is added to a word ending in *y* preceded by a consonant.

*Suffixes not beginning with* i
ninety          ninetieth
happy           happiness

*Suffixes beginning with* i
forty           fortyish

---

## 36—26    WORDS SPELLED IN MORE THAN ONE WAY

---

**_DO_**    type words spelled in more than one way according to the preferred style of your employer. If there is no preference, use the most popular and current spelling of the medical term. The first column depicts the most common spelling.

| | | | |
|---|---|---|---|
| aneurysm | aneurism | | |
| cesarean | cesarian | caesarean | caesarian |
| curet | curette | | |
| disk | disc | | |
| dysfunction | disfunction | | |
| fontanel | fontanelle | | |
| leukocyte | leucocyte | | |
| venipuncture | venepuncture | | |

# 37

# Symbols

# 37 Symbols

## INTRODUCTION

Symbols are just another form of abbreviation. Most standard symbols are available on the typewriter and word processing font menus. (See also Chapter 1, Rule 1–21.)

**_DO_**   know the technical symbols in your specialty area. Avoid the use of abbreviations in records where they are inappropriate. See Chapter 1 for help with abbreviations and Chapter 22 for help with numbers.

## 37—1   ABBREVIATIONS, SYMBOLS, AND NUMBERS

**_DO_**   spell out the symbol abbreviation when it is used alone, not in association with a number.

What is the degree of difference between the two? (not °)

**DON'T**   use a period after a symbol unless the symbol is at the end of a sentence.

**_DO_**  use symbols only when they occur in immediate association with a number or another abbreviation.

| | |
|---|---|
| 8 × 3 | eight by three |
| 4–5 | four to five |
| #3-0 | number three oh |
| 2+ | two plus |
| Vision: 20/20 | vision is twenty-twenty |
| 6/day | six per day |
| diluted 1:10 | diluted one to ten (a ratio) |
| at −2 | at minus two |
| 60/40 | sixty over forty |
| Grade IV/V | grade four over five |
| nocturia × 2 | nocturia times two |
| T&A | tonsillectomy and adenoidectomy |
| 25 mg/hr | twenty-five milligrams per hour |
| limited by 45% | limited by forty-five percent |
| 35 mg% | thirty-five milligrams percent |
| 30°C | thirty degrees Celsius |
| 99°F | ninety-nine degrees Fahrenheit |
| BP: 100/80 | blood pressure is one hundred over eighty |

**_DO_**  use figures when numbers are used *directly* with symbols, words, or abbreviations.

| | |
|---|---|
| 1+ protein | one plus protein |
| 2% | two percent |
| 75 ml/kg/24 hours | seventy-five milliliters per kilogram per twenty-four hours |
| the BUN is 45 mg% | the "bee you en" is forty-five milligrams percent |
| 99°F | ninety-nine degrees Fahrenheit |
| $10 (not $10.00) | ten dollars |
| 63 cents (not 63¢ or $.63) | sixty-three cents |
| #14 Foley or No. 14 Foley | number fourteen Foley |

# 37 Symbols

## 37—2 AMPERSAND (&) SYMBOL

**_DO_**  use the ampersand (&) symbol in phrases containing abbreviations separated by *and*. There is no space before or after the ampersand.

I&D
D&C
L&W

## 37—3 APOSTROPHE (') SIGN

See Chapter 3, *Apostrophe.*

## 37—4 ARROW (→) SIGN

**_DO_**  use an arrow when illustrating from–to in a table.

## 37—5 AT (@) SYMBOL

**_DO_**  use the at (@) symbol in informal business communications.

Order 24 syringes @ $1.50 each. (a memo)

## 37—6    CARDIOLOGIC SYMBOLS AND ABBREVIATIONS

***DO***     use cardiologic symbols and abbreviations to express electrocardiographic results.

The P waves are slightly prominent in $V_1$ to $V_3$. (or $V_1$–$V_3$) (or V1–V3)

It is not clear whether it contains a U-wave.

The QRS complexes are normal, as are the ST segments.

There are T wave inversions in LI, aVL, and V1–4 and −/+ T in V5.

***NOTE.*** *Please remember to use a lower-case "r" and apostrophe when typing rSR' (pronounced RSR prime). See Rule 3–5.*

## 37—7    CENT(¢) SIGN

See also Chapter 23, Rule 23–14.

**DON'T**     use symbols for less than whole dollar amounts.

Please give her the 35 cents change. (correct)
Please give her the 35¢ change. (incorrect)
Please give her the $0.35 change. (incorrect)

# 37 SYMBOLS

## 37—8 CHARTING SYMBOLS

**_DO_** use the following symbols when typing chart notes in medical records.

| | |
|---|---|
| * | birth |
| c̄, /c, w/ | with |
| s̄, /s, w/o | without |
| c̄c, c̄/c | with correction (eyeglasses) |
| s̄c, s̄/c | without correction (eyeglasses) |
| + | positive |
| − | negative |
| ō | negative |
| Ⓛ | left |
| Ⓡ | right |
| Rx | recipe, take |
| ℥ | ounce |
| ʒ | dram |
| ♂ | male |
| ♀ | female |
| μ | micron |
| ± | negative or positive; indefinite |
| > | greater than |
| < | lesser than |

## 37—9 CHEMICAL SYMBOLS

**_DO_** use Arabic numerals with chemical symbols. They may be typed on the same line, super- or subscript.

I-131 _or_ iodine 131 _or_ $^{131}$I

**DON'T** use periods or hyphens within chemical symbols or compounds. (See Chapter 22, Table 22–1, _Symbols for Chemical Elements and Radioactive Pharmaceuticals._)

$CO_2$  K  Na  $O_2$  $H_2O$

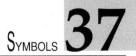

## 37—10    COLON (:) SIGN

See Chapter 5, *Colon.*

## 37—11    COMMA (,) SIGN

See Chapter 6, *Comma.*

## 37—12    DASH (—) SIGN

See Chapter 8, *Dash.*

## 37—13    DEGREE (°) SIGN

**DON'T**     use the degree (°) symbol in describing temperature if
the word degree is not dictated or is not represented
on your keyboard.

Temperature: 36C. (correct)
Temperature: 36°C. (also correct)

## 37—14    DIACRITICAL ( ` ´ ^ ~ ) MARKS

**DO**    underscore foreign expressions that are not considered part of the English language.

**DO**    use quotation marks to set off translations of foreign expressions.

**DO**    use diacritical marks on proper names.

Ramón Valenzuela
Esmé Manasson

**DO**    use diacritical marks on some, but not all, foreign words.

à la carte
à la mode
bête noire
Büngner's band
cause célèbre
cul-de-sac (no marks required)
fiancé (male) ; fiancée (female)
maître d'hôtel
matinee (no marks required)
melee (no marks required)
Mönckeberg's arteriosclerosis
pâté
puree (no marks required)
résumé
Röntgen or roentgen rays
tête-à -tête
Türk's cell
vis-à-vis

## 37—15    DOLLAR ($) SIGN

See also Chapter 22, Rule 22–14.

**_DO_**     use the dollar sign and figures to express amounts of money.

The patient's outstanding balance is $250. (correct)

The patient's outstanding balance is $250.00. (incorrect to use period and zeros when expressing whole dollar amounts)

## 37—16    EQUAL (=) SIGN

**_DO_**     use an equal sign for indicating the sum of.

24 + 50 = 74

## 37—17    EXCLAMATION POINT

See Chapter 13, *Exclamation Point.*

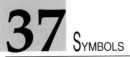

---

## 37—18 FEET (') SIGN

See also Chapter 21, *Metric System*

**_DO_**    use the ' symbol for foot and " symbol for inches if desired in technical typing and tables.

ft *or* ' (do not punctuate)
The patient is 5 ft 7 in. tall. (correct)
The patient is 5' 7" tall. (correct)

**DON'T**    pluralize this symbol or use punctuation marks with it (unless a word is formed when unpunctuated).

---

## 37—19 GREATER THAN (>) AND LESSER THAN (<) SIGNS

See Rule 37–8.

---

## 37—20 GREEK LETTERS

**_DO_**    use symbols for Greek letters if your equipment provides them. Otherwise, type out the English translation of the letter.

a (alpha)    ß (beta)    Ω (omega)    π (pi)    λ (lambda)

---

## 37—21 HYPHEN (-) AND WORD DIVISION

See Chapter 15, *Hyphen Use and Word Division.*

## 37—22     INCHES SIGN OR DITTO (") MARKS

**_DO_**      use the " symbol for inches if desired in technical typing and tables.

The patient is 5' 7" in height.

## 37—23     MINUS (–) OR PLUS (+) SIGNS

**_DO_**      use a minus sign for indicating the loss of.

**_DO_**      use plus (+) and minus (–) signs to designate the strength of a response or reaction, as well as expressing the Rhesus blood factor as Rh positive (Rh+) or Rh negative (Rh–).

Rh positive *or* Rh +
blood type O negative *or* blood type O–
knee jerks 3+ or knee jerks +++

**NOTE.** *When the phrase "plus or minus" is dictated, it may be typed as ± or +/–.*

## 37—24     NUMBER (#) SYMBOL

**_DO_**      use the number symbol with an arabic number for sizes of instruments or sutures. The symbol is preferred but may be replaced by the abbreviation *No.* When the word "number" is not dictated, you may choose whether to use the symbol # or the abbreviation *No.*

A #22 French Malecot Silastic suprapubic tube was placed in the anterior bladder dome.

The skin was closed using #4-0 Prolene interrupted vertical mattress sutures.

**DON'T** use the number symbol to indicate pounds (#) after a numeral.

> She weighed 110 pounds. (correct)
> She weighed 110 #. (incorrect)

*DO* use a symbol rather than the spelled-out word when it occurs in immediate association with a number (see Rule 22–26).

> #3-0    number three oh (dictated)

## 37—25    PARENTHESES ( )

See Chapter 23, *Parentheses.*

## 37—26    PERCENT (%) SIGN

*DO* use the percent sign or spell out the word *percent* when a number accompanies the word. There is no space between the number and the percent sign.

> 75%    1.2%    0.20%    5 percent

What is the percentage of difference between the two? (not %)

**DON'T**    use simple fractions with percent.

> 45 1/2 percent (incorrect)
> 45 1/.2% (incorrect)
> 45.5% (correct)

## 37—27    PERIOD (.)

See Chapter 25, *Period and Decimal Point.*

## 37—28    PLURALS

***DO***    use an apostrophe to form the plurals of symbols by adding 's to the singular.

> %'s    &'s    $'s    +'s

## 37—29    PLUS (+) SIGN

See Rule 37–23.

## 37—30    POUND (#) SIGN

See Rule 37–24.

# 37 SYMBOLS

## 37—31 PROOFREADING SYMBOLS

See Chapter 28, Figure 28–1.

## 37—32 QUESTION MARK (?)

See Chapter 29, *Question Mark.*

**DO** use a question mark at the end of a direct question.

Will you please return in three months for a re-examination?

**DO** use a question mark to express doubt within a sentence.

Dr. Fritz Coleman graduated from Notre Dame University in 1977 (?).

## 37—33 QUOTATION (" ")MARKS

See Chapter 30, *Quotation Marks.*

## 37—34 REFERENCE BOOKS FOR SYMBOLS

See Rules 31–1 and 31–2 for abbreviation and symbol dictionaries.

## 37—35   ROMAN NUMERALS

See also Chapter 22, Rule 22–21.

**DON'T**   use a type font that is sans serif (e.g., Chicago) because the capital letter **I** needed for Roman numerals looks like the number one.

*DO*   use Roman numerals to describe the twelve cranial nerves, the EKG limb leads, and the EEG cranial leads.

> Cranial nerves II-XII were intact.
> Cranial nerves II to XII were intact.
> Cranial lead I was not responding properly.
> The EKG limb lead III was disconnected.

*DO*   use Roman numerals with typical non-counting or non-mathematical listings. By tradition in medicine these include the following:

| | |
|---|---|
| Type | type I hyperlipoproteinemia |
| | type II diabetes mellitus |
| Factor | missing Factor VII (blood factor) |
| Stage | Stage II carcinoma |
| | Stage I coma |
| | lues II (secondary syphilis) |
| | Billroth I (first stage of a surgery) |
| Phase | Phase II clinical trials |
| Class | Class II malignancy |
| | cardiac status: Class IV |
| Grade | Grade II systolic murmur |
| Technique | Coffee technique III |
| pregnancy and delivery | Gravida II Para II Abortion O |
| with the Greek alphabet | alpha II |
| fractures | Le Fort I fracture |

# 37 Symbols

<u>**DO**</u>  use Roman numerals for major divisions in an outline (see Figure 20–9).

## ROMAN NUMERAL TABLE

| Figure | Roman Numeral | Figure | Roman Numeral |
|--------|---------------|--------|---------------|
| 1 | I | 40 | XL |
| 2 | II | 50 | L |
| 3 | III | 60 | LX |
| 4 | IV | 70 | LXX |
| 5 | V | 80 | LXXX |
| 6 | VI | 90 | XC |
| 7 | VII | 100 | C |
| 8 | VIII | 200 | CC |
| 9 | IX | 300 | CCC |
| 10 | X | 400 | CD |
| 11 | XI | 500 | D |
| 12 | XII | 600 | DC |
| 13 | XIII | 700 | DCC |
| 14 | XIV | 800 | DCCC |
| 15 | XV | 900 | CM |
| 16 | XVI | 1000 | M |
| 17 | XVII | 1500 | MD |
| 18 | XVIII | 1900 | MCM |
| 19 | XIX | 2000 | MM |
| 20 | XX | 5000 | V |
| 30 | XXX | 10,000 | X |

*NOTE.  A line over a Roman numeral multiplies the value by 1000.*

## 37—36   SEMICOLON (;)

See Chapter 32, *Semicolon.*

## 37—37    SLASH, BAR, DIAGONAL, OR SLANT (/) LINE

See Chapter 34, *Slash*.

## 37—38    SPACING WITH SYMBOLS AND NUMBERS

See also Chapter 22, Rule 22–22.

***DO***     type the following symbols directly in front of or directly following the number they refer to with no spacing.

+, =, %, #, $, °, @, &, −, /

***DO***     space each side of the × that takes the place of the word *times* or the word *by*.

## 37—39    SYMBOLS WITH ABBREVIATIONS

***DO***     use the ampersand (&) symbol in phrases containing abbreviations separated by *and*. There is no space before or after the ampersand.

I&D
D&C
L&W

**DO**    spell out the symbol abbreviation when it is used alone, not in association with a number.

What is the degree of difference between the two? (not °)

**DO**    use a symbol in preference to the spelled out word when they occur in immediate association with a number.

| | |
|---|---|
| 8 × 3 | eight by three |
| 4–5 | four to five |
| #3-0 | number three oh |
| 2+ | two plus |
| Vision: 20/20 | vision is twenty-twenty |
| 6/day | six per day |
| diluted 1:10 | diluted one to ten (a ratio) |
| at −2 | at minus two |
| 60/40 | sixty over forty |
| Grade IV/V | grade four over five |
| nocturia − 2 | nocturia times two |
| T&A | tonsillectomy and adenoidectomy |
| 25 mg/hr | twenty-five milligrams per hour |
| limited by 45% | limited by forty-five percent |
| 35 mg% | thirty-five milligrams percent |
| 30°C | thirty degrees Celsius |
| 99°F | ninety-nine degrees Fahrenheit |
| BP: 100/80 | blood pressure is one hundred over eighty |

**DON'T**    use the degree symbol (°) in describing temperature if the word degree is not dictated or is not represented on your keyboard.

Temperature: 36 C. (correct)
Temperature: 36°C. (also correct)

**DON'T** use simple fractions with percent.

> 45 1/2 percent (incorrect)
> 45 1/2% (incorrect)
> 45.5% (correct)

## 37—41    TIMES (×) OR MULTIPLIED BY SYMBOL

*DO* use the symbol × for **times** followed by a space and then the Arabic number.

> He has had nocturia × 2.

*DO* use the symbol × for **by** to express dimensions.

> The cervical stump measures 2 × 3 × 3 cm.

## 37—42    UNKNOWN (X, Y, Z) SYMBOLS

*DO* use an X symbol to denote the unknown in an abbreviation, sentence, word, or phrase. Y and Z are also used as symbols for unknown quantities or qualities.

> X marks the spot.
> fragile X chromosome
> x-ray or X-ray (in German it is X-strahlen)

> *NOTE.* *This symbol is also used to delete or obliterate.*

**DO**   use an X symbol to substitute for a group of letters when using an abbreviation.

Dx (diagnosis), Tx or Rx (treatment or prescription), Hx (history),
pedestrian Xing or railroad Xing (crossing)

# 38

# TIME

## 38—1 EVEN TIME OF DAY WRITTEN ALONE

**DO** spell out the even time of the day when written with or without *o'clock* or without *a.m.* or *p.m.*

The staff meeting is scheduled to begin at *three.*
He is due at *nine* this evening.
Give her an appointment for *two* o'clock.
She was seen as an emergency at *a quarter past ten.*

## 38—2 HOURS AND MINUTES/TIME WITH A.M AND P.M.

**DO** use figures to express the time of day with *a.m.* or *p.m.* or when both hours and minutes are expressed alone.

Office hours are from 10 a.m. to noon. Your appointment is for 11:30.

451

# 38 Time

**DON'T**  use the colon and double zeros for even periods of time.

Office hours are from 10:00 to noon. (incorrect)
Office hours are from 10 to noon. (correct)

**DON'T**  Use the expression *o'clock* with *a.m.* or *p.m.*

surgery scheduled for 3 o'clock p.m. (incorrect)
surgery scheduled for three o'clock. (correct)
surgery scheduled for 3 p.m. (correct)
surgery scheduled for three. (correct)

## 38—3  MIDNIGHT AND NOON

**DON'T**  use **a.m.** or **p.m.** with 12. You may use the figure 12 with the word *noon* or *midnight* or use the words alone without the figure 12.

We close the office at 12 noon.
My shift is over at midnight.

## 38—4  MILITARY TIME

***DO***  use figures without a colon when writing the military time of day.

0315    (zero three fifteen — 3:15 a.m.)
1200    (twelve hundred hours — noon)
1400    (fourteen hundred hours — 2 p.m.)
1630    (sixteen thirty — 4:30 p.m.)

Surgery began at precisely 16:32. (incorrect)
Surgery began at precisely 1632. (correct)

*NOTE. a.m., p.m., and o'clock are not used with military
time.*

## 38—5    PERIODS OF TIME

*DO*        write out numbers to express **periods of time** when
            the number is less than ten; when the number is over
            ten, use the figure.

            She is to return in follow-up in three months' time.

            The medical supply invoice is marked "net 30 days."

## 38—6    TIME IN POSSESSIVE CASE

*DO*        use an apostrophe to show possession of time.

            return in one month's time
            convalescence of three weeks' duration

## 38—7    CIRCULAR SURFACE EXPRESSED AS "O'CLOCK"

   Although unrelated to the time of day, the location of lesions,
injections, and incision sites on round anatomic surfaces, such as
the breast or the eye, are often expressed by referring to the face of
a clock.

# 38

***DO***

use the expression **o'clock** to refer to points on a circular surface, and use figures with *o'clock*.

The sclera was incised at about the 3 o'clock area.

The cyst was in the left breast, just below the nipple, between 4 and 5 o'clock.

Then 1:2 ml of 1% lidocaine was injected at the 4 o'clock and 8 o'clock positions.

# 39

# Underlining

# And

# Italics

## 39—1    ABBREVIATIONS

**DO**   underscore abbreviations for special emphasis.

In the following report, be sure to type p.<u>m</u>. in lower-case letters.

## 39—2    ARTISTIC WORKS

**DO**   use an underscore when typing titles of books, magazines, pamphlets, long poems, movies, plays, musicals, paintings, and other literary and artistic works. Titles of minor literary works are placed within quotation marks (see Chapter 30, *Quotation Marks*).

Mrs. Lee made it a point to see the painting of the Mona Lisa when visiting the Louvre Museum in Paris, France.

A Chorus Line was the longest running musical on Broadway.

## 39—3    BIOLOGIC NAMES

**DO**    underscore formal taxonomic names for a genus, species, subspecies, or variety in typing a manuscript for publication. If the genus name is abbreviated, this general rule should be followed.

The urinary infection was caused by Pseudomonas aeruginosa.

A common organism of uncomplicated urinary infections is E. coli.

## 39—4    DEFINITIONS

**DO**    underscore or put in quotes words that are defined or referred to.

The insured is known as a subscriber or, in some insurance programs, a member.

## 39—5    EMPHASIS

**_DO_**    underscore or put in quotes words or phrases for spe-
cial emphasis or to place emphasis on a task or com-
mand.

Dr. Johnson always mispronounces the word bruit.

Please "sterilize" these instruments immediately.

## 39—6    FOOTNOTES

See also Chapter 18, *Manuscripts.*

**_DO_**    type an underscore 2 inches long to separate footnotes
from the main text. The underscore line should be 1
line below the last line of text, beginning at the left
margin.

> _____
>
> 1. Marcy O. Diehl and Marilyn T. Fordney, Medi-
> cal Typing and Transcribing Techniques and Proce-
> dures, W. B. Saunders Company, Philadelphia, 1984,
> p. 72.

## 39—7    FOREIGN EXPRESSIONS

**_DO_**    underscore foreign expressions that are not con-
sidered part of the English language. Quote marks are
used to set off translations of foreign expressions.

It was kind of you to pick up Mr. Henry from the hospital, <u>muchas gracias</u>. (Meaning "thank you.")

In the large intestine, there is a 2½ inch area, which forms the cul-de-sac known as the cecum. (no underlining since cul-de-sac is part of the English language)

## 39—8 ITALIC TYPE FOR PRINTED MATERIAL

***DO***

use an underscore in typed material to indicate italic type in printed material.

Code numbers represent diagnostic and therapeutic <u>procedures</u> on medical billing statements and insurance forms.

## 39—9 LEGAL CITATIONS

***DO***

underscore legal case names referred to in text. The *v.* or *vs.* may or may not be underscored, depending on the employer's preference.

<u>Allen v. Levine</u>
<u>Allen v. Levine</u>
<u>Allen vs. Levine</u>

## 39—10    LITERARY WORKS

**_DO_**     use an underscore when typing titles of published books, magazines, pamphlets, long poems, movies, plays, musicals, paintings, and other literary and artistic works. Place titles of chapters, sections, and other subdivisions of a published work within quotation marks (see Chapter 30, Rule 30–4).

According to an article in <u>New Woman,</u> real estate investment is future financial protection for the career woman.

## 39—11    NAMES OF VEHICLES

**_DO_**     underscore, type with initial caps, or italicize individual names given to vehicles.

Dr. Barry returned on the cruise ship, the S.S. <u>Royal Viking.</u>
*or*
Dr. Barry returned on the cruise ship, the S.S. Royal Viking.

Dr. and Mrs. Wertlake have a Mercedes-Benz named *Otto*.

## 39—12    PLACEMENT OF UNDERSCORING

**_DO_**     underscore each word individually only when it is used as an individual word. Generally, underscore each expression as a unit.

As an expression: <u>Respondeat superior</u> means "Let the master answer."

As individual words: <u>Res, ipsa,</u> and <u>loquitur</u> are Latin words.

**_DO_** underline headings in medical reports if it is the preferred format of your employer. (See Chapter 19, *Medical Reports.*)

## 39—13 PUNCTUATION

**DON'T** underline punctuation marks following the underlined material.

**DON'T** break the underscore to skip punctuation within the underscored material.

Do you have the book by Mary Louise Gilman entitled <u>One Word, Two Words, Hyphenated?</u> in your library?

Have you read that excellent article in the <u>Star Free Press,</u> "The AIDS Epidemic"?

**DON'T** underscore a possessive or plural ending that is added on to an underscored word.

There are too many buts in that paragraph.

The <u>New York Times</u>'s editorial gave the projected population of the United States for the year 2000.

## 39—14   TITLES OF PUBLISHED WORKS

**_DO_**   use an underscore when typing titles of published books, computer programs (software), journals, magazines, pamphlets, long poems, movies, plays, musicals, paintings, and other literary and artistic works. Place titles of chapters, sections, and other subdivisions of a published work within quotation marks (see Chapter 30, Rule 30–4).

Esther just finished reading The Wizard of Oz.

**_NOTE._**   _Titles of journals (e.g.,_ J. Inf. Dis.) _that appear in reference lists or bibliographies do not have to be underscored._

# 40

## VITAE

## FORMAT

## AND

## PREPARATION

## INTRODUCTION

The physician's curriculum vitae, or professional profile, is used in the following situations:

1. As evidence of the expertise of a physician who is testifying as an expert witness
2. To introduce a physician who has been invited as a guest speaker or who is appearing on television

3. To seek employment in a hospital staff position or apply for a faculty appointment at a teaching hospital
4. To obtain a research grant from a federal or funding agency
5. To determine if an institution is complying with state and voluntary agency requirements for physicians who have certain positions in hospitals
6. To obtain agency accreditation for residency training programs

## 40—1  ACADEMIC CREDENTIALS

See Rule 40–7.

## 40—2  AFFILIATIONS

**DO**   list membership in professional associations, showing category of membership, name of the organization, date membership began followed by a hyphen and the word *present* if membership is continuing. Double-space between entries if listing more than one organization.

Member, New York State Medical Society, 1980–present

Fellow, American College of Physicians 1980–present

## 40—3  BIBLIOGRAPHIES OF PUBLICATIONS AND ABSTRACTS

See Rule 40–19.

## 40—4  BOARD CERTIFICATION

**_DO_**  type the name of the board where the physician received certification, followed by the year certification was received. Double space between entries if listing more than one specialty area, beginning each entry on a separate line.

American Board of Orthopaedic Surgery, 1982

## 40—5  BOARD ELIGIBILITY

**_DO_**  type the name of the board examination for which the physician is eligible to sit.

American Board of Internal Medicine —
Infectious Diseases

## 40—6  CONTINUATION SHEETS

**_DO_**  begin numbering with the second sheet as page 2 in the upper right corner.

## 40—7  EDUCATION

**_DO_**  list chronologically all medical and academic degrees held by the physician by typing the college or university from which the undergraduate degree was earned and then the school from which the medical degree was earned. Double-space between these two groups of information.

**DO**     type the name of the college or university followed by the name of the city and state where the school is located.

**DO**     type the kind of degree earned and the years of attendance or the year the degree is granted.

*NOTE.*  *A sub-subheading under this category might be* Postdoctoral Study.

George Washington University, School of Medicine, Washington, D.C.
M.D., 1980

## 40—8     FACULTY APPOINTMENTS

**DO**     type the academic rank (assistant, associate, full professor, lecturer) and the name of the medical school or college. One line below, type the city and state of the school and the years of appointment. Double space between entries if there is more than one appointment.

Associate Professor, UCLA School of Medicine
Los Angeles, California, 1980–85

## 40—9     FELLOWSHIP

**DO**     type the name of the hospital where fellowship training was completed, followed by the name of the city and state where the institution is located. One line below, type the kind of fellowship training, the word *Fellowship*, and the dates of fellowship training.

Westlake Community Hospital, Westlake Village, California
Plastic Surgery Fellowship, 1981–83

## 40—10    FORMAT (Fig. 40–1)

**_DO_**    use 8 1/2" × 11" white or off-white bond paper typed leaving 1-1/2" margins all around.

**_DO_**    use a high-quality photocopying process (offset or laser printing), and keep the original document in a plastic protector so it is not given away by mistake.

**DON'T**    include personal information (hobbies or children's names) other than the physician's name, office and/or home address, and telephone number.

> **OPTIONAL.**    *Birthdate, place of birth, marital status.*

**DON'T**    overuse underlining and capitalization.

**_DO_**    spell out names of organizations and agencies.

**_DO_**    spell out titles.

**_DO_**    proofread the curriculum vitae carefully for spelling and punctuation.

**_DO_**    update the physician's curriculum vitae every two or three months.

**Figure 40–1.** Illustration of a curriculum vitae.

---

CURRICULUM VITAE

Josephine B. Wells, M. D.

PERSONAL HISTORY

Business Address:   329 West Main Street, Suite 430
Weston, PA 19016

Telephone:   (805) 890-5399

EDUCATION

| 1980 | New York State University, New York, New York B.S., Biology |
| 1985 | George Washington University, Washington, D.C. M. D. with Honors |

INTERNSHIP

| 1985–86 | UCLA Medical Center, Los Angeles, California Internship (Straight Medicine) |

RESIDENCY

| 1986–87 | UCLA Medical Center, Los Angeles, California Internal Medicine Residency |

FELLOWSHIP

| 1987–89 | Cook County Hospital, Chicago, Illinois Infectious Disease Fellowship |

BOARD CERTIFICATION

| 1988 | American Board of Internal Medicine |

BOARD ELIGIBILITY

American Board of Internal Medicine —
Infectious Diseases

(continued)

---

Josephine B. Wells Curriculum Vitae (continued)    2

HONORS

| 1986 | Intern of the Year, UCLA Medical Center<br>Los Angeles, California |
|---|---|

MEDICAL LICENSURE

State of California (G027037) June 1985

MEDICAL SPECIALTY

| 1985–present | Internal Medicine |
|---|---|

PROFESSIONAL AFFILIATIONS

| 1985–present | Fellow, American College of Physicians |
|---|---|
| 1985–present | Member, California Medical Association |

STAFF APPOINTMENTS

| 1989–present | Attending Physician, Westside Medical Center<br>Los Angeles, California |
|---|---|
| 1990–present | Associate Attending Physician, Community<br>Memorial Hospital<br>Los Angeles, California |

STAFF POSITIONS

| 1990–present | Chairperson, Bioethics Committee<br>Westside Medical Center, Los Angeles,<br>California |
|---|---|

FACULTY APPOINTMENTS

| 1990–present | Assistant Professor, UCLA Medical School<br>Los Angeles, California |
|---|---|

TEACHING EXPERIENCE

| 1989–90 | Guest Lecturer, Rheumatology Course<br>UCLA Medical School<br>Los Angeles, California |
|---|---|

## 40—11    HEADING

**_DO_**  center the all-capitalized heading CURRICULUM VITAE 1-1/2" from the top of the first page. The physician's name and degree abbreviations are centered and typed two line spaces beneath the heading.

CURRICULUM VITAE
Mary T. O'Connor, M. D.

## 40—12    HONORS

**_DO_**  type the name of the award or honor and the agency giving the award. One line below, type the name of the city and state and the year the award was given. Double space between each award and honor.

Intern of the Year, New York Masonic Medical Center
New York, New York, 1984

## 40—13    INTERNSHIP (First year of postgraduate medical education)

**_DO_**  type the name of the hospital and city and state where the internship was completed. One line below, type the word _Internship_ and, in parentheses, the type (Straight Medicine or Rotating) followed by the dates of internship.

New York Masonic Medical Center, New York, New York
Internship (Straight Medicine), 1980

## 40—14    LICENSURE

**_DO_**       list license numbers for all states, giving the name of the state and the month and year the license was issued.

State of California (018-502897) June 1980

## 40—15    MILITARY SERVICE

**_DO_**       type the military position held by the physician and the branch of service. One line below, type the city and state where he or she was stationed and the years of service.

Major, U. S. Army, Chief of Surgery
Bangkok, Thailand, 1981–1983

## 40—16    PERSONAL DATA

**DON'T**    include personal information (hobbies or children's names) other than the physician's name, office and/or home address, and telephone number.

> **_OPTIONAL._**    _Birthdate, place of birth, marital status._

## 40—17    POSTDOCTORAL TRAINING

See _Internship_, Rule 40–13, and _Residency_, Rule 40–21.

## 40—18    PROFESSIONAL TRAINING AND EXPERIENCE

**_DO_**   type the specialty of medical practice (Fig. 40–1) followed by the years of service. One line below, type the city and state where the practice is located. Double space between entries if the physician has more than one practice. This section should be in chronological order. List the current practice and work back to residency and internship.

## 40—19    PUBLICATIONS (Fig. 40–2)

**_DO_**   list three categories (journals, books and other monographs, and meeting presentations) on separate sheets of paper in chronological order, according to their dates of publication or presentation.

**_DO_**   list the authors' names in the same order as they appear in the publication.

Pankow, C. W. and Cherrick, H. Carcinoma of the tongue. J. Oral Surg. 1981; 20:193–96.

**DON'T**   underline any part of a citation except the genus and species of micro-organisms and Latin words.

Vincent, R. and Derby, K. Quantitative testing for <u>Escherichia coli</u>. J. Path. 1984; 23:234–36.

**Figure 40–2.** Illustration of three pages — bibliographies of publications, books and other monographs, and meeting presentations.

## BIBLIOGRAPHIES OF PUBLICATIONS

### JOURNALS

Wells, Josephine B. , Richie, R. F. Nucleolar antigen specific for anti-nucleolar antibody in sera of patients with systemic rheumatic disease. J. Inf. Dis. 1985; 10:135–37.

Wells, Josephine B., Messert, B. Asymptomatic gonorrhea in women: Diagnosis, natural course and prevalence. N. Engl. J. Med. 1985; 14:150–52.

### BOOKS AND OTHER MONOGRAPHS

Wells, Josephine B., Sanders, B., The Menopause, F. A. Davis, Philadelphia, 1987.

### MEETING PRESENTATIONS

| | |
|---|---|
| February 1981 | "Gold Pays Off in Arthritis"<br>UCLA School of Medicine<br>Lecture to Senior Residents in<br>Internal Medicine |
| October 1982 | "Drug Prevents Calcium Stones"<br>State Medical College<br>Lecture to Senior Pharmacy<br>Students |

## 40—20    RESEARCH PROJECTS

**_DO_**   type the name of the project, and the name of the company, hospital, or agency for which the physician is conducting research. Type the status of the research project (ongoing, completed, or expected completion date) one line below and the beginning and ending dates of the project. Double-space between entries if there is more than one research project.

Electromagnetophoresis, National Institutes of Health
Completed research, 1980–1990

## 40—21    RESIDENCY

**_DO_**   type the name of the hospital where residency train-ing was completed, followed by the name of the city and state where the hospital is located. One line below, type the name of the specialty followed by the word _Residency_ and the dates of residency training.

Cook County Medical Center, Miami, Florida
Internal Medicine Residency, 1986–87

## 40—22    STAFF APPOINTMENTS

**_DO_**    type the category of the staff appointment (senior at-
tending physician, associate attending physician, consulting physician, courtesy physician, and so forth)
followed by the name of the institution. One line
below, type the name of the city and state where the
hospital is located followed by the years in which the
appointment was held. Double space between entries
if there is more than one appointment.

Senior Attending Physician, Bethesda Hospital
Bethesda, Maryland, 1980–present

## 40—23    STAFF POSITIONS

**_DO_**    type the name of the position held and the years ser-
ved. One line below, type the name of the hospital followed by the city and state where located. If the
physician served on a committee, list the name of the
committee.

*NOTE.    Staff appointment is an initial appointment to
the hospital staff, and staff position is subsequent to that.*

Chairman, Bioethics Committee, 1988–present
Vista Medical Center, Cleveland, Ohio

## 40—24    SUBHEADINGS

**_DO_**        type major subheadings flush with the left margin. Single-space each cluster of data beneath the subheadings. Double-space between the subheadings and the first line of the date. Double- or triple-space between subheads depending on the available space. Subheadings may be in all capital letters with or without underscoring or in capital and lower-case letters and underscored. (See Fig. 40–1.)

**_DO_**        use the following categories:

Staff appointments
Staff positions
Faculty appointments
Practice experience
Teaching experience
Research projects
Journals
Books and other monographs
Meeting presentations (optional)

## 40—25    TEACHING EXPERIENCE

**_DO_**        type the name of the teaching program, the name of the hospital, the city and state where located, and the years the physician was associated with the program. If the physician was a lecturer, so indicate.

Pain Control, UCLA School of Medicine
Los Angeles, California, 1984–85

# Wᴏʀᴅ

---

## FINDER

---

## INTRODUCTION

The following are some common examples of how English and medical terms sound and a clue as to how they are spelled to help you locate them in the medical dictionary. If you cannot find a word when you look it up, refer to this table and use another combination of letters that has the same sound. For example: Look up the sound "n" in the word *pneumonia*. Notice that the "n" sound as in "no" could be spelled *cn, gn, kn, mn, nn, pn*. Thus, you have some clues as to how to locate the word in the dictionary. (See also Chapter 36, *Spelling.*)

| If the Sound Is Like . . . | Try the Spelling as in . . . | Examples |
|---|---|---|
| a in fat | ai | pl<u>ai</u>d |
| | al | h<u>al</u>f |
| | au | dr<u>au</u>ght |
| | | |
| a in sane | ai | p<u>ai</u>n |
| | ao | g<u>ao</u>l |
| | au | g<u>au</u>ge |
| | ay | p<u>ay</u>, x-r<u>ay</u>, T<u>ay</u>-Sachs |
| | ue | s<u>ue</u>de |
| | ie | p<u>ie</u>dra |
| | ea | br<u>ea</u>k |
| | ei | v<u>ei</u>n |

| If the Sound Is Like . . . | Try the Spelling as in . . . | Examples |
|---|---|---|
| | eigh | weigh |
| | et | sachet |
| | ey | they, peyote |
| a in care | ai | air, clairvoyant |
| | ay | prayer |
| | e | there |
| | ea | wear |
| | ei | their |
| a in father | au | aural, auricle, auscultation |
| | e | sergeant |
| | ea | heart |
| a in ago | e | agent |
| | i | sanity |
| | o | comply |
| | u | focus |
| | iou | vicious |
| aci in acid | acy | acystia |
| ak | ac | accident |
| | ach | achromatic |
| | acr | acromegaly |
| ark | arch | archicyte |
| b in big | bb | rubber |
| | pb | cupboard |
| bak sound in back | bac | bacteremia |
| bee | by | presbyopia |
| ch in chin | c | cello |
| | Cz | Czech |
| | tch | stitch |
| | ti | question |
| | tu | denture, fistula |

| If the Sound Is Like . . . | Try the Spelling as in . . . | Examples |
|---|---|---|
| d in do | dd | pu<u>dd</u>le |
| | ed | call<u>ed</u> |
| die | di | <u>di</u>agnosis, <u>di</u>arrhea |
| dis | dis | <u>dis</u>charge |
| | dys | <u>dys</u>pnea |
| dew | deu | <u>deu</u>teropathy |
| | dew | <u>dew</u>lap |
| | du | <u>du</u>ra |
| e in get | a | <u>a</u>ny |
| | ae | <u>ae</u>sthetic |
| | ai | s<u>ai</u>d |
| | ay | s<u>ay</u>s |
| | e | <u>e</u>dema |
| | ea | h<u>ea</u>d |
| | ei | h<u>ei</u>fer |
| | eo | l<u>eo</u>pard |
| | ie | fr<u>ie</u>nd |
| | oe | r<u>oe</u>ntgen |
| | u | b<u>u</u>rial |
| e in equal | ae | h<u>ae</u>moglobin |
| | ay | qu<u>ay</u> |
| | ea | l<u>ea</u>n |
| | ee | fr<u>ee</u> |
| | ei | dec<u>ei</u>t |
| | eo | p<u>eo</u>ple |
| | ey | k<u>ey</u> |
| | i | hem<u>i</u>cardia |
| | ie | s<u>ie</u>ge |
| | oe | am<u>oe</u>ba |
| | y | tracheotom<u>y</u> |
| e in here | ea | <u>ea</u>r |
| | ee | ch<u>ee</u>r |
| | ei | w<u>ei</u>rd |
| | ie | b<u>ie</u>r |

| If the Sound Is Like . . . | Try the Spelling as in . . . | Examples |
|---|---|---|
| ek | ec | lectotype, eczema |
| | ek | ekphorize |
| er in over | ar | liar |
| | ir | elixir |
| | or | author, labor |
| | our | glamour |
| | re | acre |
| | ur | augur |
| | ure | measure |
| | yr | zephyr |
| eri, ere, aire | ery | erythrocyte, erythema |
| ex | ex | extravasation |
| | x | x-ray |
| f in fine | ff | cliff |
| | gh | laugh, slough |
| | lf | half |
| | ph | physiology, prophylactic |
| fizz | phys | physical |
| floo, flu | flu | fluoride, fluoroscopy |
| g in go | gg | egg |
| | gh | ghost |
| | gu | guard |
| | gue | prologue |
| gli in glide | gly | glycemia |
| grew | grou | group |
| guy (also see jin) | gy | gynecomastia |
| h in hat | g | Gila monster |
| | j | San Joaquin Valley fever |
| | wh | who, whooping cough |

| If the Sound Is Like . . . | Try the Spelling as in . . . | Examples |
|---|---|---|
| he | he | <u>he</u>matoma |
| | hae (British spelling) | <u>hae</u>matology |
| hi in high | hy | <u>hy</u>drocele |
| i in it | a | us<u>a</u>ge |
| | e | <u>E</u>nglish |
| | ee | b<u>ee</u>n |
| | ia | carr<u>ia</u>ge |
| | ie | s<u>ie</u>ve |
| | o | w<u>o</u>men |
| | u | b<u>u</u>sy |
| | ui | b<u>ui</u>lt |
| | y | lar<u>y</u>ngeal, n<u>y</u>stagmus |
| i in kite | ai | gu<u>ai</u>ac |
| | ay | <u>ay</u>e |
| | ei | h<u>ei</u>ght, m<u>ei</u>osis |
| | ey | <u>ey</u>e |
| | ie | t<u>ie</u> |
| | igh | n<u>igh</u> |
| | is | <u>is</u>land of Langerhans |
| | uy | b<u>uy</u> |
| | y | m<u>y</u>ograph |
| | ye | r<u>ye</u> |
| ik or ick | ich | <u>ich</u>thyosis |
| ink | inc | <u>inc</u>ubator |
| j in jam | d | gra<u>d</u>ual |
| | dg | ju<u>dg</u>e |
| | di | sol<u>di</u>er |
| | dj | a<u>dj</u>ective |
| | g | re<u>g</u>ister, fun<u>g</u>i |
| | ge | ven<u>ge</u>ance |
| | gg | exa<u>gg</u>erate |
| jin | gyn | <u>gyn</u>ecology |

| If the Sound Is Like . . . | Try the Spelling as in . . . | Examples |
|---|---|---|
| k in keep | c | eczema |
| | cc | account |
| | ch | chronic, tachycardia |
| | ck | tack |
| | cq | acquire |
| | cu | biscuit |
| | lk | walk |
| | qu | liquor |
| | que | plaque |
| key | che | chemotherapy |
| | chy | ecchymosis |
| ko | cho, co | cholecyst, colon |
| kon | chon | chondroma |
| | con | condyloma |
| kw sound in quick | ch | choir |
| | qu | quintuplet |
| l in let | ll | call |
| | sl | isle |
| la in lay | lay | layette |
| | le | lei |
| lack | lac | lacrimal |
| loo | leu | leukocyte |
| | lew | lewisite |
| m in me | chm | drachm |
| | gm | phlegm |
| | lm | balm |
| | mb | limb |
| | mm | hammer toe |
| | mn | hymn |

| If the Sound Is Like . . . | Try the Spelling as in . . . | Examples |
|---|---|---|
| mass | mac | macerate |
| mix | myx | myxedema |
| n in no | cn | cnemial |
| | gn | gnathic |
| | kn | knife |
| | mn | mnemonic |
| | nn | tinnitus |
| | pn | pneumonia |
| ng in ring | ngue | tongue |
| new | neu | neurology |
| | pneu | pneumococcus |
| o in go | au | mauve |
| | eau | beau |
| | eo | yeoman |
| | ew | sew |
| | oa | foam |
| | oe | toe |
| | oh | ohm |
| | oo | brooch |
| | ou | shoulder |
| | ough | dough |
| | ow | row |
| o in long | a | all |
| | ah | Utah |
| | au | fraud |
| | aw | thaw |
| | oa | broad |
| | ou | ought |
| off | oph | exophthalmos, ophthalmology |
| oi in oil | oy | boy |
| oks | occ | occiput |
| | ox | oxygen |

| If the Sound Is Like . . . | Try the Spelling as in . . . | Examples |
|---|---|---|
| oo in tool | eu | le<u>u</u>kemia |
| | ew | dr<u>ew</u> |
| | o | m<u>o</u>ve |
| | oe | sh<u>oe</u> |
| | ou | gr<u>ou</u>p |
| | ough | thr<u>ough</u> |
| | u | r<u>u</u>le, t<u>u</u>laremia |
| | ue | bl<u>ue</u> |
| | ui | br<u>ui</u>se |
| oo in look | o | w<u>o</u>lffian |
| | ou | w<u>ou</u>ld |
| | u | p<u>u</u>ll, tubercu<u>u</u>losis |
| ow in out | ou | m<u>ou</u>th |
| | ough | b<u>ough</u> |
| | ow | cr<u>ow</u>d |
| p in put | pp | ha<u>pp</u>y |
| pack | pach | myopa<u>ch</u>ynsis, pa<u>ch</u>yderma |
| pi in pie | py | nephro<u>py</u>osis |
| r in red | rh | <u>rh</u>abdocyte |
| | rr | be<u>rr</u>y |
| | rrh | ci<u>rrh</u>osis, hemo<u>rrh</u>oid |
| | wr | <u>wr</u>ong, <u>wr</u>ist |
| re in repeat | rhe | <u>rhe</u>ostosis |
| | ri | mala<u>ri</u>a |
| | rrhe | oto<u>rrhe</u>a |
| rew | rheu | <u>rheu</u>matism |
| | rhu | <u>rhu</u>barb |
| rom | rho | <u>rho</u>mboid |
| rye | rhi | <u>rhi</u>noplasty |

| If the Sound Is Like . . . | Try the Spelling as in . . . | Examples |
|---|---|---|
| s in sew | c | cyst, foci |
| | ce | rice |
| | ps | psychology |
| | sc | sciatic, viscera |
| | sch | schism |
| | ss | miss |
| | sth | isthmus |
| sh in ship | ce | ocean |
| | ch | chancre |
| | ci | facial |
| | s | sugar |
| | sch | Schwann's cell |
| | sci | fascia |
| | se | nauseous |
| t in tea | pt | pterygium, ptosis |
| zh sound in azure | ge | garage, massage, curettage |
| | s | vision |
| | si | fusion |
| | zi | glazier |
| zi (rhymes with sigh) | x | xiphoid, xanthoma |
| | zy | zygoma, zygote, enzyme |
| zz | ss | scissors |
| | zz | buzz |

As an additional spelling aid, here is a group of letter combinations that can cause problems when you are trying to locate a word.

| If You Have Tried . . . | Then Try . . . |
|---|---|
| pre | per, pra, pri, pro, pru |
| per | par, pir, por, pur, pre, pro |
| is | us, ace, ice |
| ere | ear, eir, ier |
| wi | whi |

# 41 WORD FINDER

| If You Have Tried . . . | Then Try . . . |
|---|---|
| we | whe |
| zi | xy |
| cks, gz | x |
| tion | sion, cion, cean, cian |
| le | tle, el, al |
| cer | cre |
| si | psi, ci |
| ei | ie |
| dis | dys |
| ture | teur |
| tious | seous, scious |
| air | are, aer |
| ny | gn, n |
| ance | ence |
| ant | ent |
| able | ible |
| fizz | phys |

## $Z_{IP}$

## CODES

---

## INTRODUCTION

The Zone Improvement Plan (ZIP) is a system of numerical codes consisting of five or nine digits to be written or typed on envelopes to expedite the delivery of mail. If it is omitted from the envelope, the correspondence will be delayed.

## 42—1    ABBREVIATIONS

See also Chapter 1, *Abbreviations and Symbols,* Rule 1–20.

**_DO_**      use the two-letter state abbreviations approved by the United States Postal Service for both inside and envelope addresses. See Figure 1–1 in Chapter 1, page 4, for abbreviations for the United States and Canadian provinces and territories.

**DON'T**    use the abbreviations without the city name and ZIP Code.

# 42 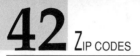ZIP CODES

## 42—2    ADDRESS FORMAT

See also Chapter 2, *Address Formats for Letters and Forms of Address*, Rules 2–3 and 2–11 and Chapter 11, *Envelope Preparation*, Rule 11–2.

**_DO_**    leave 1 to 3 spaces between the state name and the ZIP Code.

## 42—3    CANADIAN POSTAL CODE

**_DO_**    place the Canadian code on a line by itself or after the abbreviation for the province (separated by a two-character space).

| | | |
|---|---|---|
| Dr. Thomas B. Larchmont | *or* | Dr. Thomas B. Larchmont |
| 1858 Haversley Court | | 1858 Haversley Court |
| Vancouver, British Columbia | | Vancouver, BC V3J 1W1 |
| V3J 1W1 | | |

## 42—4    CITY, STATE, AND ZIP CODE

**_DO_**    type the city, state, and ZIP code on one line, after the street address.

New York, NY 10158    *or*    New York, NY 10158-0012

## 42—5    ENVELOPE PREPARATION

See Chapter 11, *Envelope Preparation*, Rule 11–2.

## 42—6    REFERENCES

**_DO_**    obtain a missing ZIP code by calling your local post office, visiting a local library, or purchasing a ZIP code directory at a stationery or book store. A book entitled _ZIP + 4 Code State Directory_ is available from the United States Postal Service.

## 42—7    SENTENCE

**_DO_**    insert a comma after the street address and after the city when typing an address in a sentence. There is one space between the state and ZIP code.

Dr. Hancock's new address will be 3300 West Main Street, Suite 505, Miami, Florida 33144-2728, but this will not be effective until June 1.

## 42—8    WORD DIVISION

**_DO_**    divide between the city and the state or between the state and the ZIP code. If the city or state contains two or more words, divide between the words.

New York, / New York 10004

_or_

New York, New York / 10004

_or_

New / York, New York 10004

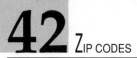

**_DO_**     use the nine-digit ZIP code to expedite and reduce mailing costs when sending by bulk mail.

San Francisco, CA 94120-7168     San Diego, CA 92109-3602
Portland, OR 97204-2628          New York, NY 10005-4101

# APPENDIX

## Common Medical Homonyms

The following words are commonly encountered in medical transcription. You will notice that they are in alphabetical sequence with the homonyms indented below each word. Phonetics are shown and the stress point of the word is capitalized. Abbreviated definitions are listed so that you do not have to refer to your medical dictionary unless you wish a more detailed meaning.

abduction — ab-DUK-shun
  *addiction*
  *adduction*
  *subduction*

A drawing away from the midline.

aberration — ab"er-A-shun
  *abrasion*
  *erasion*
  *erosion*
  *operation*

Deviation from the usual course.

abrasion — ah-BRA-shun
  *aberration*
  *erasion*
  *erosion*
  *operation*

Denudation of skin.

absorption — ab-SORP-shun
*adsorption*
*sorption*

The uptake of substances into tissues.

addiction — ah-DIK-shun
*abduction*
*adduction*

Dependence on a drug or some habit.

adduction — ah-DUK-shun
*abduction*
*addiction*

A drawing toward the midline.

adherence — adh-HER-ens
*adhered to*
*adherent*
*adherents*

The act or quality of sticking to something.

adsorption — ad-SORP-shun
*absorption*
*sorption*

To collect in condensed form on a surface.

affect — af-FEKT
*effect*

To have an influence on; the feeling experienced in connection with an emotion.

afferent — AF-er-ent
*aberrant*
*efferent*

Conveying toward a center.

alveolar — al-VE-o-lar
*alveolate*
*alveoli*
*alveolus*
*alveus*
*alvus*
*areolar*

Pertaining to an alveolus.

alveoli — al-VE-o-li
*alveolar*
*alveolate*
*alveolus*
*alveus*
*alvus*
*areolar*

Plural of alveolus.

alveolus — al-VE-o-lus
*alveolar*
*alveolate*
*alveoli*
*alveus*
*alvus*
*areolar*

A small saclike dilatation.

alveus — AL-ve-us
*alveolar*
*alveolate*
*alveoli*
*alveolus*
*alvus*
*areolar*

A trough or canal.

alvus — AL-vus
  *alveolar*
  *alveolate*
  *alveoli*
  *alveolus*
  *alveus*
  *areolar*

The abdomen with its contained viscera.

amenorrhea — ah-men"o-RE-ah
  *dysmenorrhea*
  *menorrhagia*
  *menorrhea*
  *metrorrhagia*

Abnormal stoppage of the menses.

antiseptic — an"ti-SEP-tik
  *asepsis*
  *aseptic*
  *sepsis*
  *septic*

Preventing decay or putre-faction.

aphagia — ah-FA-je-ah
  *abasia*
  *aphakia*
  *aphasia*

Abstention from eating.

aphakia — ah-FA-ke-ah
  *aphagia*
  *aphasia*

Absence of the lens of the eye.

aphasia — ah-FA-ze-ah
  *abasia*
  *aphagia*
  *aphakia*

Loss of the power of expression by speech, writing, or signs.

apposition — ap"o-ZISH-un
  *opposition*

The placing of things in juxtaposition or proximity.

arrhythmia — ah-RITH-me-ah
  *erythema*
  *eurhythmia*

Variation from the normal rhythm of the heart beat.

arteriosclerosis — ar-te"re-o-skle-RO-sis
  *arteriostenosis*
  *atherosclerosis*

A disease characterized by thickening and loss of elas-ticity of arterial walls.

arteriostenosis — ar-te"re-o-ste-NO-sis
  *arteriosclerosis*
  *atherosclerosis*

The narrowing or diminution of the caliber of an artery.

atherosclerosis — ath"er-o"skle-RO-sis
  *arteriosclerosis*
  *arteriostenosis*

Deposits of yellowish plaques containing cholesterol and lipoid material formed on the inside of the arteries.

aural — AW-ral
  *aura*
  *ora*
  *oral*

Pertaining to or perceived by the ear.

auscultation — aws"kul-TA-shun
*oscillation*
*oscitation*
*osculation*

The act of listening for sounds within the body.

bare — ber
*bear*

Naked.

border — BOR-der
*boarder*
*quarter*

A rim, margin, or edge.

bowel — BOW-el
*bile*
*vowel*

The intestine.

breath — breth
*breadth*

The air taken in and expelled by the expansion and contraction of the thorax.

breathe — brēth
*breed*

To take air into the lungs and let it out again.

bronchoscopic — brong"ko-SKOP-ik
*proctoscopic*

Pertaining to bronchoscopy or to the bronchoscope.

bruit — brwe, broot
*brute*

A sound or murmur heard in auscultation.

calculous — KAL-ku-lus
*calculus*
*caliculus*
*callous*
*callus*

Pertaining to, of the nature of, or affected with calculus.

calculus — KAL-ku-lus
*calculous*
*caliculus*
*callous*
*callus*

Any abnormal stony mass or deposit formed in the body.

callous — KAL-us
*calculous*
*calculus*
*callus*
*talus*

A hardened, thickened place on the skin. (adj.)

callus — KAL-us
*calculous*
*calculus*
*callous*
*talus*

A hardened, thickened place on the skin; new growth of bone cells at a fracture site. (noun)

cancellous — KAN-sĕ-lus
*cancellus*
*cancerous*

Of a reticular, spongy, or lattice-like structure.

cancellus — kan-SEL-us
*cancellous*
*cancerous*

Any structure arranged like a lattice.

cancer — KAN-ser
*canker*
*chancre*

Malignant tumor.

cancerous — KAN-ser-us
*cancellous*
*cancellus*

Pertaining to cancer.

canker — KANG-ker
*cancer*
*chancre*

Ulceration, chiefly of
the mouth and lips.

carbuncle — KAR-bung-kl
*caruncle*
*furuncle*

A cluster of boils; furuncles.

carpus — KAR-pus
*carpal*
*corpus*

The wrist.

caruncle — KAR-ung-kl
*carbuncle*
*furuncle*

A small fleshy eminence,
whether normal or
abnormal.

chancre — SHANG-ker
*cancer*
*canker*

The primary sore of syphilis.

cirrhosis — sir-RO-sis
*cillosis*
*psilosis*
*sclerosis*
*serosa*
*xerosis*

A degenerative disease of the
liver.

coarse — kors
*course*
*force*

Not fine or microscopic;
rough or crude.

contusion — kon-TU-zhun
*concussion*
*confusion*
*convulsion*

A bruise.

cord — kord
*chord*
*cor*

Any long, rounded, flexible
structure. Also spelled chord
and chorda.

corneal — KOR-ne-al
*cranial*

Pertaining to the cornea of the
eye.

corpus — KOR-pus
*carpus*
*copious*
*core*
*corps*
*corpse*

Body.

cranial — KRA-ne-al
*corneal*

Pertaining to the cranium
(skull).

cytology — si-TOL-o-je
  *psychology*
  *sitology*

The study of cells.

diaphysis — di-AF-ĭ-sis
  *apophysis*
  *diastasis*
  *diathesis*
  *epiphysis*

Shaft of a long bone.

diathesis — di-ATH-ĕ-sis
  *diaphysis*
  *diastasis*

A predisposition to certain diseases.

dilatation — dil-ah-TA-shun
  *dilation*

A dilated condition or structure.

dilation — di-LA-shun
  *dilatation*

The process of dilating or becoming dilated.

dysphagia — dis-FA-je-ah
  *dysbasia*
  *dyscrasia*
  *dysphasia*
  *dysplasia*
  *dyspragia*

Difficulty in swallowing.

dysphasia — dis-FA-ze-ah
  *dysbasia*
  *dyscrasia*
  *dysphagia*
  *dysplasia*
  *dyspragia*

Impairment of the faculty of speech.

dysplasia — dis-PLA-se-ah
  *dysbasia*
  *dyscrasia*
  *dysphagia*
  *dysphasia*
  *dyspragia*

Abnormality in development of tissue or body parts.

dyspragia — dis-PRA-je-ah
  *dysphagia*
  *dysphasia*
  *dysplasia*

Painful performance of any function.

dyspraxia — dis-PRAK-se-ah
  *dystaxia*

Partial loss of ability to perform coordinated acts.

ecchymosis — ek"i-MO-sis
  *achymosis*
  *echinosis*
  *echomosis*

A bruise.

effect — e-FEKT
  *affect*
  *defect*

The result; to bring about.

efferent — EF-er-ent
  *aberrant*
  *afferent*

Conveying away from a center.

elicit — e-LIS-it
  *illicit*
To cause to be revealed; to draw out.

embolus — EM-bo-lus
  *bolus*
  *embolism*
  *thrombus*
A blood clot carried in the bloodstream.

endemic — en-DEM-ik
  *ecdemic*
  *epidemic*
  *pandemic*
A disease native to a particular region.

enervation – en"er-VA-shun
  *denervation*
  *innervation*
Lack of nervous energy; removal or section of a nerve.

enteric — en-TER-ik
  *icteric*
Pertaining to the small intestine.

epidemic — ep"i-DEM-ik
  *ecdemic*
  *endemic*
The rapid spreading of a contagious disease.

erythema — er"i-THE-mah
  *arrhythmia*
  *erythremia*
  *eurhythmia*
Redness of the skin due to a variety of causes.

eschar — ES-kar
  *a scar*
  *escharotic*
  *scar*
A slough produced by a thermal burn or by gangrene.

everted — e-VER-ted
  *inverted*
Turned outward.

facial — FA-shal
  *basal*
  *fascial*
  *faucial*
  *racial*
Pertaining to the face.

fascial — FASH-e-al
  *facial*
  *falcial*
  *fascia*
  *fashion*
  *faucial*
Pertaining to fascia.

fauces — FAW-sēz
  *facies*
  *feces*
  *foci*
  *fossa*
  *fossae*
The throat.

fecal — FE-cal
  *cecal*
  *fetal*
  *focal*
  *thecal*
Pertaining to or of the nature of feces.

fetal — FE-tal
*fatal*
*fecal*

Pertaining to a fetus.

flexor — FLEK-sor
*flexure*

Any muscle that flexes a joint.

flexure — FLEK-sher
*flexor*

A bent position of a structure or organ.

fundi — FUN-di
*fungi*

Plural of fundus, a bottom or base.

furuncle — FU-rung-k'l
*carbuncle*
*caruncle*

A boil.

gastroscopy — gas-TROS-ko-pe
*gastrostomy*
*gastrotomy*

Inspection of the stomach with a gastroscope.

gastrostomy — gas-TROS-to-me
*gastroscopy*
*gastrotomy*

Artificial opening into the stomach.

gavage — gah-VAHZH
*lavage*
*garage*

Feeding by stomach tube.

glands — glands
*glans*

Groups of cells that secrete or excrete material not used in their metabolic activities.

glans — glanz
*glands*

Latin for gland.

hypercalcemia — hi"per-kal-SE-me-ah
*hyperkalemia*
*hypocalcemia*

An excess of calcium in the blood.

hyperinsulinism — hi"per-IN-su-lin-izm"
*hypoinsulinism*

Excessive secretion of insulin by the pancreas; insulin shock.

hyperkalemia — hi"per-kah-LE-me-ah
*hypercalcemia*
*hyperkinemia*
*hypokalemia*

Abnormally high potassium concentration in the blood.

hypertension — hi"per-TEN-shun
*Hypertensin*
*hypotension*

High blood pressure.

hypocalcemia — hi"po-kal-SE-me-ah
*hypercalcemia*
*hyperkalemia*

Reduction of the blood calcium below normal.

hypoinsulinism — hi"po-IN-su-lin-izm
*hyperinsulinism*

Deficient secretion of insulin by the pancreas.

hypokalemia — hi"po-ka-LE-me-ah
*hypercalcemia*
*hyperkinemia*
*hyperkalemia*

Abnormally low potassium concentration in the blood.

hypotension — hi"po-TEN-shun
*hypertension*

Low blood pressure.

icteric — ik-TER-ik
  *enteric*
  *mycteric*

Pertaining to or affected with jaundice.

ileum — IL-e-um
  *ilium*

Part of the small intestine.

ilium — IL-e-um
  *ileum*

The flank bone or hip bone.

illicit — i-LIS-it
  *elicit*

Illegal.

infarction — in-FARK-shun
  *infection*
  *infestation*
  *infraction*
  *injection*

The formation of an infarct.

infection — in-FEK-shun
  *infarction*
  *infestation*
  *inflection*
  *inflexion*
  *in flexion*
  *injection*

Invasion of the body by pathogenic micro-organisms.

infestation — in-fes-TA-shun
  *infarction*
  *infection*
  *injection*

Invasion of the body by small invertebrate animals, such as insects, mites, or ticks.

injection — in-JEK-shun
  *infarction*
  *infection*
  *infestation*
  *ingestion*

Act of forcing a liquid into a part or an organ.

innervation — in"er-VA-shun
  *enervation*

The distribution of nerves to a part.

insulin — IN-su-lin
  *inulin*

Protein formed by the islet cells of Langerhans in the pancreas.

inulin — IN-u-lin
  *insulin*

A vegetable starch.

inverted — in-VERT-ed
  *everted*

Turned inside out or upside down.

keratitis — ker"ah-TI-tis
  *keratiasis*
  *keratosis*
  *ketosis*

Inflammation of the cornea.

keratosis — ker"ah-TO-sis
  *keratitis*
  *keratose*
  *ketosis*

Any horny growth, such as a wart or a callosity.

ketosis — ke-TO-sis
  *keratitis*
  *keratosis*

Abnormally high concentration of ketone bodies in the body tissues and fluids.

laceration — las"er-A-shun
  *maceration*
  *masturbation*

Act of tearing; wound made by tearing.

lavage — lah-VAHZH
  *gavage*

The irrigation or washing out of an organ.

lipoma — li-PO-mah
  *fibroma*
  *lipomyoma*
  *lymphoma*

A benign tumor composed of mature fat cells.

lithotomy — lith-OT-o-me
  *lithotony*

Incision of an organ for removal of stone.

lithotony — lith-OT-o-ne
  *lithotomy*

Creation of an artificial vesical fistula that is dilated to extract a stone.

liver — LIV-er
  *livor*
  *sliver*

A large gland of dark-red color in the upper part of the abdomen on the right side.

livor — LIV-or
  *liver*

Discoloration.

lymphoma — lim-FO-mah
  *lipoma*

Any neoplastic disorder of the lymphoid tissue.

maceration — mas"er-A-shun
  *laceration*
  *masturbation*

The softening of a solid by soaking.

mastitis — mas-TI-tis
  *mastoiditis*

Inflammation of the mammary gland, or breast.

mastoiditis — mas"toi-DI-tis
  *mastitis*

Inflammation of the mastoid antrum and cells.

masturbation — mas"tur-BA-shun
  *laceration*
  *maceration*

Production of orgasm by self- manipulation of the genitals.

menorrhagia — men"o-RA-je-ah
  *menorrhea*
  *metrorrhagia*

Excessive uterine bleeding at menstruation.

menorrhea — men"o-RE-ah
  *amenorrhea*
  *dysmenorrhea*
  *menorrhagia*
  *metrorrhagia*

The normal discharge of the *menses*.

metacarpal — met"ah-KAR-pal
  *metatarsal*

Pertaining to the metacarpus.

metastasis — me-TAS-tah-sis
*metaphysis*
*metastases (plural)*
*metastasize*
*metastatic*

The transfer of disease from one site to another not directly connected with it.

metastasize — me-TAS-tah-size
*metastases*
*metastasis*
*metastatic*

To form new foci of disease in a distant part by metastasis.

metastatic — met"ah-STAT-ik
*metastases*
*metastasis*
*metastasize*

Pertaining to metastasis.

metatarsal — met"ah-TAR-sal
*metacarpal*

Pertaining to the metatarsus.

metrorrhagia — me"tro-RA-je-ah
*menorrhagia*
*menorrhea*

Uterine bleeding at irregular intervals, sometimes being prolonged.

mucoid — MU-koid
*mucor*
*mucosa*
*mucosal*

Resembling mucin.

mucosa — mu-KO-sah
*mucosal*
*mucosin*
*mucous*
*mucus*

A mucous membrane.

mucosal — mu-KO-sal
*mucosa*
*mucous*
*mucus*

Pertaining to the mucous membrane.

mucous — MU-kus
*mucosa*
*mucosal*
*mucus*

The adjective that means pertaining to mucus.

mucus — MU-kus
*mucosa*
*mucosal*
*mucous*

The noun that means a viscid watery secretion of mucous glands.

myogram — MI-o-gram
*myelogram*

A recording or tracing mode with a myograph.

necrosis — ne-KRO-sis
*narcosis*
*nephrosis*
*neurosis*

Death of tissue.

nephrosis — ne-FRO-sis
*necrosis*
*neurosis*
*tephrosis*

Any disease of the kidney.

neurosis — nu-RO-sis
*necrosis*
*nephrosis*
*urosis*

Disorder of psychic or mental constitution.

obstipation — ob"sti-PA-shun
*constipation*
*obfuscation*

Intractable constipation.

oral — O-ral
*aura*
*aural*

Pertaining to the mouth.

oscillation — os"i-LA-shun
*auscultation*
*oscitation*
*osculation*

A backward and forward motion; vibration.

oscitation — os"i-TA-shun
*auscultation*
*excitation*
*oscillation*
*osculation*

The act of yawning.

osculation — os"ku-LA-shun
*auscultation*
*escalation*
*oscillation*
*oscitation*

To kiss; to touch closely.

palpation — pal-PA-shun
*palliation*
*palpillation*
*palpitation*

The act of feeling with the hand.

palpitation — pal"pi-TA-shun
*palliation*
*palpation*
*papillation*

Regular or irregular rapid *action of the heart.*

parasthenia — par"as-THE-ne-ah
*paresthesia*

A condition of organic tissue causing it to function at abnormal intervals.

paresthesia — par"es-THE-ze-ah
  *pallesthesia*
  *parasthenia*
  *paresthenia*

An abnormal sensation, such as burning or prickling.

parietitis — pah-ri"ĕ-TI-tis
  *parotitis*
  *parotiditis*

Inflammation of the wall of an organ.

parotiditis — pah-rot"ĭ-DI-tis
  *parietitis*
  *parotitis*

Inflammation of the parotid gland.

parotitis — par"o-TI-tis
  *parietitis*
  *parostitis*
  *parotiditis*

Inflammation of the parotid gland.

parous — PA-rus
  *Paris*
  *pars*
  *porous*

Having brought forth one *living offspring.*

pedicle — PED-ĭ-k'l
  *medical*
  *particle*
  *peduncle*
  *pellicle*

A footlike or stemlike structure.

perineal — per"i-NE-al
  *pectineal*
  *peritoneal*
  *peroneal*

Pertaining to the perineum.

perineum — per"i-NE-um
  *peritoneum*

The region at the lower end of the trunk between the thighs.

peritoneum — per"i-to-NE-um
  *perineum*

The serous membrane lining the abdominal walls.

peroneal — per"o-NE-al
  *pectineal*
  *perineal*
  *peritoneal*
  *peronia*

Pertaining to the fibula or outer side of the leg.

pleural — PLOOR-al
  *plural*

Pertaining to the pleura.

prostate — PROS-tāt
  *prostrate*

A gland in the male which surrounds the neck of the bladder and the urethra.

prostrate — PROS-trāt
  *prostate*
Lying flat, prone, or supine.

psychology — si-KOL-o-je
  *cytology*
  *sitology*
The science dealing with the mind and with mental and emotional processes.

pyelonephrosis — pi"e-lo-nĕ-FRO-sis
  *pyonephrosis*
Any disease of the kidney and its pelvis.

pyonephrosis — pi"o-nĕ-FRO-sis
  *pyelonephrosis*
Suppurative destruction of the parenchyma of the kidney.

pyrenemia — pi"rĕ-NE-me-ah
  *pyoturia*
  *pyuria*
The presence of nucleated red cells in the blood.

pyuria — pi-U-re-ah
  *paruria*
  *pyorrhea*
  *pyoturia*
  *pyrenemia*
The presence of pus in the urine.

radical — RAD-ĭ-kal
  *radicle*
Directed to the source of a morbid process, as radical surgery.

radicle — RAD-ĭ-k'l
  *radical*
Any one of the smallest branches of a vessel or nerve.

recession — re-SESH-un
  *resection*
The act of drawing away or back.

reflex — RE-fleks
  *efflux*
  *reflux*
A reflected action; an involuntary muscular movement.

reflux — RE-fluks
  *efflux*
  *reflex*
A backward or return flow.

resection — re-SEK-shun
  *recession*
Excision of a portion of an organ or other structure.

rhonchi — RONG-kī
  *bronchi*
  *ronchi*
Plural of rhonchus, a rattling in the throat; a dry, coarse rale.

scar — skahr
  *a scar*
  *eschar*
  *scarf*
A mark remaining after the healing of a wound.

scirrhous — SKIR-us     Pertaining to a hard
  *cirrhosis*               cancer.
  *cirrus*
  *scirrhus*
  *sclerous*
  *serious*
  *serous*
scirrhus — SKIR-us     Scirrhous carcinoma.
  *cirrhosis*
  *cirrus*
  *scirrhous*
  *sclerous*
  *serious*
  *serous*
sedentary — SED-en-ter"e     Sitting habitually.
  *sedimentary*
sedimentary — sed-ĭ-MEN-ter-e     Of, or having the nature
  *sedentary*               of, or containing sediment.
separation — sep-ah-RA-shun     Break; division; gap.
  *suppression*
  *suppuration*
sepsis — SEP-sis     The presence in the blood
  *antiseptic*              of pathogenic microor-
  *asepsis*                ganisms or their toxins.
  *aseptic*
  *septic*
  *threpsis*
septic — SEP-tik     Due to decomposition by
  *antiseptic*              microorganisms.
  *asepsis*
  *a septic*
  *aseptic*
  *sepsis*
  *septal*
  *septile*
  *skeptic*
serosa — se-RO-sah; se-RO-zah     Any serous membrane
  *cirrhosis*              (tunica mucosa); tunica
  *xerosia*                serosa; the chorion.

| | |
|---|---|
| serous — SE-rus<br>  *cirrus*<br>  *scirrhous*<br>  *scirrhus*<br>  *sclerous*<br>  *sera*<br>  *serious*<br>  *serose* | Pertaining to serum. |
| sight — sīt<br>  *cite*<br>  *cyte*<br>  *side*<br>  *site*<br>  *slight* | The act of seeing; a thing seen. |
| stasis — STA-sis<br>  *bases*<br>  *basis*<br>  *station*<br>  *status*<br>  *staxis* | A stoppage of the flow of blood. |
| staxis — STAK-sis<br>  *stasis* | Hemorrhage. |
| stroma — STRO-mah<br>  *soma*<br>  *stoma*<br>  *struma*<br>  *trauma* | The supporting tissue of an organ. |
| struma — STROO-mah<br>  *stoma*<br>  *stroma* | Goiter. |
| suppression — sŭ-PRESH-un<br>  *separation*<br>  *suppuration* | The sudden stoppage of a secretion, excretion, or normal discharge. |
| suppuration — sup"u-RA-shun<br>  *separation*<br>  *suppression*<br>  *susurration* | The formation of pus. |
| sycosis — si-KO-sis<br>  *psychosis* | A disease marked by in-flammation of the hair follicles; a kind of ulcer on the eyelid. |
| tenia — TE-ne-ah<br>  *taenia*<br>  *Taenia*<br>  *tinea* | A flat band or strip of soft tissue. |

thenar — THE-nar
*femur*
*thinner*

The mound on the palm at the base of the thumb.

thrombus — THROM-bus
*embolus*

A blood clot which remains at the site of formation.

tinea — TIN-e-ah
*linea*
*linear*
*taenia*
*Taenia*
*tenia*

Ringworm.

trachelotomy — tra"ke-LOT-o-me
*tracheophony*
*tracheotomy*

The surgical cutting of the uterine neck.

tracheophony — tra"kě-OF-o-ne
*trachelotomy*
*tracheotomy*

A sound heard in auscultation over the trachea.

tracheotomy — tra"ke-OT-o-me
*trachelotomy*
*tracheophony*

Incision of the trachea through the skin and muscles of the neck.

tympanites — tim"pah-NI-těz
*tympanitis*

Distention of the abdomen due to gas or air in the intestine or in the peritoneal cavity.

tympanitis — tim"pah-NI-tis
*tenonitis*
*tinnitus*
*tympanites*

Inflammation of the middle ear.

ureter — u-RE-ter
*urethra*
*urethral*
*ureteral*

The tube which conveys the urine from the kidney to the bladder.

ureteral — u-RE-ter-al
*ureter*
*urethra*
*urethral*

Pertaining to the ureter.

urethra — u-RE-thrah
*ureter*
*ureteral*

The canal conveying urine from the bladder to the outside of the body.

urethral — u-RE-thral
*ureter*
*ureteral*
*urethra*

Pertaining to the urethra.

urethrorrhagia — u-re"thro-RA-je-ah A flow of blood from
  *ureterorrhagia* the urethra.
uterus — u-ter-us The womb.
  *ureter*
  *urethra*
  *urethral*
vagitis — va-JI-tis Inflammation of the vagal
  *vagitus* nerve.
vagitus — vah-JI-tus The cry of an infant.
  *vagitis*
vagus — VA-gus The tenth cranial nerve.
  *valgus*
valgus — VAL-gus Bent outward, twisted,
  *vagus* as in knock-knee
  *varus* (genu valgum).
  *vastus*
variceal — var"ĭ-SE-al Pertaining to a varix, an
  *varicella* enlarged artery or vein.
varicella — var"ĭ-SEL-ah Chickenpox.
  *variceal*
varicose — VAR-ĭ-kos Pertaining to a varix, an
  *verrucose* enlarged artery or vein.
  *very close*
  *very coarse*
variolar — vah-RI-o-lar Pertaining to smallpox.
  *variola*
venous — VE-nus Pertaining to the veins.
  *Venus*
Venus — VE-nus The goddess of love and
  *venous* beauty in Roman myth-
ology; the planet second
from the sun.
verrucose — VER-oo-kōs Rough; warty.
  *varicose*
  *verrucous*
  *vorticose*
verrucous — VER-oo-kus Rough; warty.
  *varicose*
  *verrucose*
  *vorticose*

vesical — VES-ĭ-kal
  *fascicle*
  *vesica*
  *vesicle*
  *vessel*

Pertaining to the bladder.

vesicle — VES-ĭ-k'l
  *fascicle*
  *vesica*
  *vesical*
  *vessel*

A small bladder or sac containing liquid.

vessel — VES-'l
  *vesical*
  *vesicle*

A tube or duct containing or circulating a body fluid.

villous — VIL-us
  *villose*
  *villus*

Shaggy with soft hairs.

villus — VI-lus
  *villose*
  *villous*

A small vascular process or protrusion.

viscera — VIS-er-ah
  *visceral*
  *viscus*

Plural of viscus.

viscus — VIS-kus
  *discus*
  *vicious*
  *viscera*
  *viscose*
  *viscous*

Any large interior organ in any one of the three great cavities of the body.

womb — wo͞om
  *wound*

The uterus.

wound — wo͞ond
  *womb*

An injury to the body caused by physical means.

xerosis — ze-RO-sis
  *cirrhosis*
  *serosa*

Abnormal dryness.

The light face numbers in this index refer to page numbers. The **boldface** numbers refer to paragraph (rule) numbers. Italics indicate figure pages and t indicates tables.

ISBN 0-7216-3798-1